Complete Conditioning for
BASEBALL

Pat Murphy
Head Baseball Coach
Arizona State University

Jeff Forney
Strength and Conditioning Coach
Arizona Diamondbacks

Human Kinetics

Library of Congress Cataloging-in-Publication Data

Murphy, Pat, 1958-
   Complete conditioning for baseball / Pat Murphy, Jeff Forney
     p.   cm.
   ISBN 0-87322-886-3
    1. Baseball--Training.   2. Physical fitness.   I. Forney, Jeff, 1963-   II. Title.
   GV875.6.M87   1997
   796.357'07--dc21
                                              96-48333
                                                CIP
ISBN: 0-87322-886-3

Developmental Editor: Julie Rhoda; **Assistant Editor:** Sandra Merz Bott; **Editorial Assistant:** Jennifer J. Hemphill; **Copyeditor:** John Wentworth; **Proofreader:** Bob Replinger; **Graphic Designer:** Stuart Cartwright; **Graphic Artist:** Tom Roberts; **Photo Editor:** Boyd La Foon; **Cover Designer:** Jack Davis; **Photographer (cover):** Anthony Neste; **Photographer (interior):** Jeffrey Forney; **Illustrators:** Beth Young and Tim Stiles; **Printer:** United Graphics

Human Kinetics books are available at special discounts for bulk purchase. Special editions or book excerpts can also be created to specification. For details, contact the Special Sales Manager at Human Kinetics.

Printed in the United States of America   10   9   8   7   6   5

Human Kinetics
Web site: www.humankinetics.com

United States: Human Kinetics, P.O. Box 5076, Champaign, IL 61825-5076
800-747-4457
e-mail: humank@hkusa.com

Canada: Human Kinetics, 475 Devonshire Road, Unit 100, Windsor, ON N8Y 2L5
800-465-7301 (in Canada only)
e-mail: hkcan@mnsi.net

Europe: Human Kinetics, P.O. Box IW14, Leeds LS16 6TR, United Kingdom
+44 (0)113 278 1708
e-mail: humank@hkeurope.com

Australia: Human Kinetics, 57A Price Avenue, Lower Mitcham, South Australia 5062
08 8277 1555
e-mail: liahka@senet.com.au

New Zealand: Human Kinetics, P.O. Box 105-231, Auckland Central
09-309-1890
e-mail: hkp@ihug.co.nz

CONTENTS

ACKNOWLEDGMENTS

Pat Murphy would like to thank everyone involved in the making of this manuscript. Thanks to Human Kinetics for recognizing Arizona State's baseball program and the importance of baseball conditioning. Special thanks to my friend, Mack Newton, for his inspiration and guidance.

Jeff Forney would also like to thank everyone involved in the making of this manuscript. Thanks to the Arizona Diamondbacks for their support and understanding of the importance of overall baseball strength and conditioning. Special thanks to Mack Newton, who I consider not only a friend and mentor, but also a source of great inspiration. And last but not least, a very special thanks to my wife, Sandi, for first deciphering my handwriting and then helping me to type, edit, and produce this manuscript.

FOREWORD

As a Major League baseball manager, I've had the good fortune to manage some of the best players in the game. The one thing they all have in common is the solid baseball skills needed to get to the top of the game. What distinguishes the great players from the good players, aside from natural talent, is an elevated level of dedication to improving their overall game—everything from baseball skills like hitting and throwing to their strength and conditioning regimen.

When I became the manager for the Arizona Diamondbacks, I knew we had a unique opportunity to see the organization develop from the ground level. One of our main objectives was not only to get the most talented players for our Major League team, but also to establish a comprehensive program for our Minor League players, many of whom will become our future stars. Our approach to achieving this goal has included a solid strength and conditioning program, and Jeff Forney has brought just such a program to our organization.

Jeff's program isn't a generic routine for athletes of various sports altered to apply to baseball players. Rather, it is designed specifically for meeting baseball player's needs—a uniquely baseball-specific conditioning program. It takes into account the need for such skills as speed and agility in the field, as well as strength and explosive power at the plate.

Since implementing this conditioning program during our initial seasons, we've seen our players improve noticeably. By following our training program, they

- developed far more flexibility and agility,
- maintained body weight while increasing muscle mass and decreasing percent body fat,
- increased upper and lower body strength,

- enhanced explosive power, and
- gained a better awareness of the importance of conditioning in their overall baseball success.

Not only have we experienced these dramatic gains, we've also established a basis for continued improvement. This baseball-specific conditioning program—much of which is in complete conditioning for baseball—keeps the athletes interested by varying the workout routines and incorporating a variety of training tools and techniques. The workouts are designed to help you achieve the maximum amount of improvement in the minimum amount of time.

We feel we've identified a key component of our organization's success. Our conditioning program enhances our players' performance and establishes a standard that we believe is among the best in the league. You may not have access to a professional strength and conditioning coach at every training session, but you can use the information provided in *Complete Conditioning for Baseball* to help you improve your physical development and raise your overall game to a higher level.

Buck Showalter
Manager, Arizona Diamondbacks

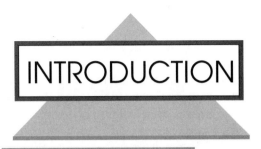

INTRODUCTION

All baseball players, from Little League through the majors, must be physically ready to perform the skills the game requires. "Ready" means different things to different people. The best players, those who go the furthest in the game and achieve the most success, don't feel ready unless they can perform the skills their position demands *to their utmost ability*. A progression of the skills necessary for baseball success can be represented by a pyramid (figure A). At the wide base of the pyramid are seasons full of games and thousands of excited athletes with various

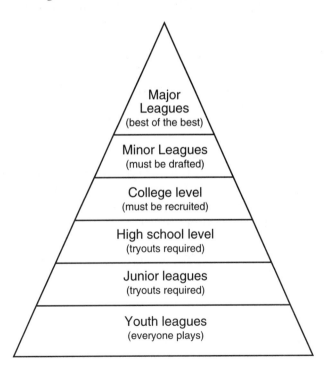

Figure A   Baseball progression pyramid.

degrees of skill and potential. As the levels progress, the pyramid narrows because fewer players have the required levels of skill, physical talent, and enthusiasm for the game to continue playing. Only a small fraction reach the top of the pyramid—the major leagues—but no matter what level of baseball you play, through proper physical training and a positive attitude, you can excel. Don't ever sell yourself short—do what it takes to reach your maximum athletic potential through total body conditioning.

Baseball coaches will tell you that what separates the best players from the rest is athletic ability. This is why such a premium is placed on the player who possesses rare physical tools, such as the combination of speed and power of Barry Bonds, the brute strength of Frank Thomas, or the great durability of Nolan Ryan. These players are not born with these skills. They were born with the capability to achieve them. If they hadn't drilled their speed, honed their strength, and built their power through hard work and proper conditioning, they would never have become the valuable players that they did. Nolan Ryan says his longevity was largely due to his strength and conditioning program. Carlton Fisk, who played in the majors well into his 40s, maintained a daily ritual of postgame strength and conditioning workouts—even after extra-inning night games.

Total body conditioning requires a combination of exercises and drills aimed at improving overall aerobic fitness, flexibility, power, and reaction time. For the baseball player, a complete conditioning program helps improve base-running speed, fielding reaction time, and speed and power at the plate or on the mound. A successful conditioning program also includes sound nutrition to help the player stay tuned up and healthy. It took a while for baseball coaches and players to embrace complete conditioning. The old school of thinking viewed conditioning in baseball as an unnecessary evil. After all, Babe Ruth hit 714 big-league homers with a beer gut, right? More recently, John Kruk won a batting title while citing his lack of conditioning and couch-potato habits. But what if the Babe and Kruk and many other players past and present worked as hard on their physical training as they did when they were playing on the field? Who knows—a healthy and conditioned Babe might have hit 1,000 homers.

The majority of today's coaches and managers know that solid methods specifically for improving baseball skills and conditioning are out there. These methods strengthen players, helping them swing the bat harder and hit the ball farther, or pitch or throw harder and faster. The player with greater speed improves his base-stealing potential and can run down more balls in the field. Increased flexibility allows a player to reach and stretch farther for those oh-so-close outs at the base. And of course, during a long season, the well-conditioned player will less likely succumb to injuries, allowing him to play at his best for the whole season. It is the player who works *smart*, not just hard, who succeeds in this game. Our goal is to help baseball players improve both physically and mentally through our complete conditioning program.

Baseball has been around a long time and is justifiably labeled America's pastime. Not until recently, however, have scientifically proven techniques and methods specifically for improving baseball become available. In this book, we will describe these methods and techniques and tell you how to apply them through drills. In chapter 1 we'll discuss the basic foundation of complete conditioning for baseball players and introduce training concepts such as periodization and specificity so you can start developing a complete training program. In chapter 2 we offer basic nutrition guidelines for baseball players—because you can't play your best if you don't fuel your body right. In chapter 3 we'll show you how to warm up and stretch prior to your workouts. The remaining chapters are then devoted to helping you develop in specific areas. Chapters 4 and 5 focus on exercises to improve your strength and power; in chapters 6 and 7, the emphasis is on increasing your speed and agility. In chapters 8, 9, and 10, we present increasingly advanced, specialized drills and exercises to continually challenge players and develop their abilities. Finally, in chapter 11, we describe sample training programs to help you tailor the information we've provided to best fit your needs.

Wherever you are currently in your game, if you apply the knowledge we pass along in these pages, you'll be ready for the next step. Good luck, work smart, and most important—have fun!

CHAPTER 1

BENEFITS OF COMPLETE CONDITIONING FOR THE BASEBALL PLAYER

Because of baseball's long tradition in this country, many ideas are slow to change regarding how baseball players should be trained. Some coaches choose to take the "safe" route of doing things the way they have always been done. Other coaches want to try something new but are reluctant to incorporate systematic training programs in fear of hindering their athletes by implementing a program based on unfounded concerns and fallacies. For example, many people still think that weight training makes baseball players bulky and limits their range of motion. This is not so—in fact, weight training the right way can improve range of motion and does not necessarily cause bulk. Of course there is much more to a good training program than just lifting weights. Our goal in this book is to help educate the baseball community on the benefits of a comprehensive and properly administered conditioning program. Over the years, we've seen many athletes enter our program weak and underdeveloped. Through conditioning, they become faster, stronger, and better all-around players. The myths and rumors you hear about training and baseball being a bad mix are simply inaccurate. We have seen far too much evidence to the contrary!

BUILDING THE FOUNDATION

When you build a house, you don't start with the roof—you first lay the foundation and then build up from there. So it goes with baseball conditioning. A good training program begins with a strong foundation phase that includes both cardiovascular fitness and muscle endurance. As you know, playing baseball requires certain levels of fitness, strength, and speed. The higher the level you achieve in these areas, the greater potential you have as a player. It's often the case that an increased level in one of the areas leads to an improvement in another. For example, to increase your speed, you need to exert more power against the ground. The ability to exert more power comes from an increase in strength. So, to increase your speed, try supplementing your wind sprints with squats and power cleans. These exercises use three times the muscle mass of any other weight-training exercise for the legs while approximating the movements used in the sprint stride. We'll discuss how this works in more detail in chapter 6. For now, let's take a quick look at the building blocks of our conditioning program: cardiovascular fitness, range of motion, strength and muscular endurance, and speed.

Cardiovascular Fitness

Basically, cardiovascular training allows you to accomplish more work with less fatigue; it leads to faster recuperation between sets, exercises, and workouts. Cardiovascular exercise fits into one of two categories: *aerobic* (with oxygen) and *anaerobic* (without oxygen). Aerobic training increases the body's demand for oxygen, which in turn adds to the workload of the heart and lungs. This kind of training gets oxygen to the muscles more efficiently, allowing them to work longer during conditioning or competition. It also works to burn excess or unnecessary body fat. Some of the more popular forms of aerobic exercise include distance running, cycling, stair climbing, and jumping rope.

Anaerobic training includes exercises that burn energy without the use of oxygen. Glycogen stored in the muscles is the primary fuel used during anaerobic exercise, which includes activities requiring short bursts (10 to 20 seconds) of energy, such as sprinting and weightlifting. These short bursts also lead to an increase in your heart workload, although not for the sustained period that aerobic exercise requires. Because baseball movements are generally short and explosive, conditioning for baseball includes much more anaerobic training than aerobic.

Range of Motion

Once we have established good cardiovascular fitness, we want to improve our range of motion, which is critical in baseball. Stretching exercises and warm-up techniques that take the muscles through a full range of motion help improve overall flexibility. We'll discuss flexibility and warm-up in detail in chapter 3.

Strength and Muscular Endurance

We stressed earlier that a sound baseball conditioning program consists of more than just weight training. However, weight training is the primary means of building the strength that helps us improve our speed, power, and agility. The key is to keep the focus on improving strength and not just bulking up. Following the guidelines provided in chapters 4 and 5, we'll help you target the essential muscles used in our game.

Speed

Speed is a measure by which all good athletes, including baseball players, are judged. A player with speed automatically possesses a weapon that separates him from a slower opponent. There is no way to defend speed except through speed itself, so if you can become quicker than the players you face, you will have an edge over them. We'll discuss speed in detail in chapter 6.

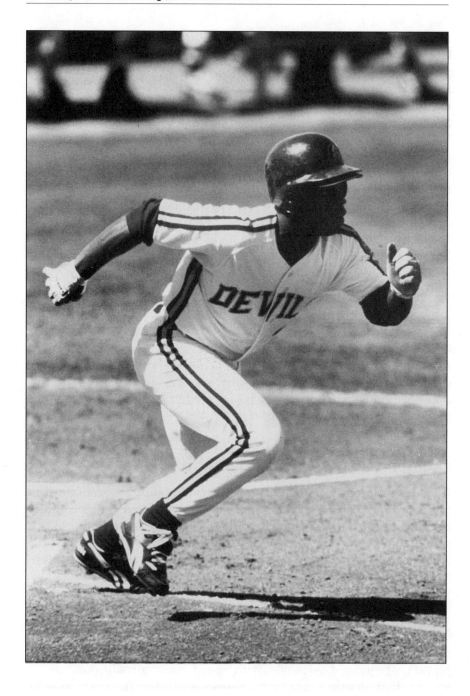

TRAINING PRINCIPLES

Knowing the areas you need to improve in and learning a few exercises that address these areas is *not* enough to design a successful conditioning program. To yield the best results, you need to know which exercises to do when and the specific ways to do them best—that is, you need to apply training principles. These principles include periodization; specificity and adaptation; and intensity, frequency, and duration.

Periodization

The success of a training program depends on the logical development of successive training sessions, or *periodization*. Unfortunately, periodization is absent from many training programs. A good coach understands the reasoning behind his or her training program and continually adjusts the program to optimize results while reducing the risk of injury and overtraining.

Periodization was developed in the Soviet Union and Eastern Europe to train high-level athletes. The theory behind periodization is to divide phases of training into small, manageable segments so that the body does not adapt to the training; this creates a gradual, planned increase in performance that peaks in time for competition. Periodization significantly reduces the risk of injury because it emphasizes a gradual increase in overall training levels.

Periodization is a systematic approach tailored for an individual or team. The training cycle can last any length of time, from a few weeks to a year. The guesswork of what kind of workout or exercise to do today is taken away, as each workout is part of a progressive, planned program. The progression from one period to the next is gradual, and as the stages come together we get our systematic linking.

A mistake commonly made when designing a workout program is to place too much stress on a player before his body can adequately tolerate it, which causes an injury. In the beginning, it is always better to err on the side of caution rather than risk injury to an athlete early and set your program back tremendously. For this reason, you should design your program with gradual increases in intensity, through periodization. Periodization as we apply it to our baseball training program consists of six standard training phases:

1. Regeneration
2. Strength

3. Power
4. Specific power
5. Preseason
6. In-season

Regeneration: All baseball players need this phase. After a long season, you need not only a physical but also a psychological renewal. This is a transition phase to our upcoming training season and also a good time for necessary surgeries and rehabilitation. The regeneration phase lasts anywhere from three to eight weeks, depending on the length of the season just completed and the physical condition of the athlete. During this time, you can have an active rest when you can participate in other sports that you enjoy at your leisure. You should try to do some type of exercise three to five times per week during this period.

Strength: This is the adjustment period after the regeneration phase or for newcomers to weight training and total conditioning. The focus here is on building overall cardiovascular fitness and light weight training. This phase includes exercises that are light in intensity, with rest between sets of one to two minutes. This phase could last two to six weeks depending on the athlete's background and fitness.

Power: This phase converts strength gains into power. This is achieved through plyometrics, speed work, and agility drills. This phase lasts five weeks.

Specific power: In this phase the focus is on developing maximum strength, sport-specific power. Strength is the key ingredient for both power and muscular endurance. During this phase, we use the heaviest amounts of weight possible. This phase lasts from two to three weeks, depending again on the fitness of the athlete or team and how much time is available.

Preseason: The goal of the preseason phase is to slowly taper off the heavy weights and training sessions to prepare for the season. This is where we begin to cut back on the intensity, frequency, and duration of the workouts. During this two-week phase we start focusing on actual baseball skills such as throwing, hitting, and fielding.

In-season: This is sometimes called the maintenance phase. Our focus now is on playing baseball. Training sessions two to three times a week during this phase are sufficient to maintain strength gains attained during the previous phases.

This brief outline of periodization is intended to give you basic training concepts. Remember to emphasize both individual and team needs. Working smarter rather than just harder is key to maximizing gains in conditioning.

Specificity and Adaptation

Specificity and *adaptation* are terms to know when you're ready to consider what exercises to include in your training program. Specificity means that the area or skill requiring improvement must be specifically trained. For example, if we're targeting speed gains, we need to implement exercises specifically aimed at improving speed—running mechanics, leg strength, stride, and so on. Adaptation as it applies to conditioning is the process of familiarizing your body systems to exercise. We want to constantly manipulate that adaptation to challenge our bodies to perform at higher levels.

Intensity, Frequency, and Duration

You are probably familiar with the terms intensity, frequency, and duration, but we want to define them here as they'll be used in this book. *Intensity* is the power output or rate of performing the work in an exercise. We can usually increase intensity by using a heavier resistance or moving the load faster. *Frequency* is the number of training sessions over a set period of time. *Duration* is the length of each session or the amount of time it takes to perform an exercise.

NEEDS ANALYSIS

To customize our conditioning program for baseball, we should make a biomechanical analysis of the sport. While determining the muscle groups used most often in our sport and targeting those muscles with specific exercises to strengthen them, we should consider the following:

1. Which muscle groups need to be trained?
2. What are the primary sites of injury for baseball?
3. Which exercises best strengthen the muscles used?
4. What individual needs of players need to be addressed?

Once you have assessed the needs of your training program, tailor the program accordingly. Here are some key points to remember when applying your program (these points will be discussed in more detail in later chapters):

1. More is not better. Don't run down your athletes. Use training cycles that allow proper rest for muscles.
2. Never teach an exercise that you can't perform or teach properly.
3. Stress the importance of mental focus. Emphasize working smarter, not just harder.
4. Stay involved. Maintain enthusiasm and avoid monotony by changing exercises to continually challenge the athlete.

EFFORT AND MENTAL FOCUS: BE LIKE CAL!

A great example of a player who has displayed and benefited from developing a great mental focus is Cal Ripken, Jr. His accomplishments as baseball's Ironman would not have been achieved without great physical *and* mental preparation. As you know by now, baseball requires a tremendous amount of mental focus. It's mind boggling that some players can stay so mentally tough throughout a long season. But others have trouble maintaining a strong mental focus. The attitude that *I'll be prepared physically and mentally and through this preparation I'll gain confidence that will help me perform better* is a great advantage for a player to have. We have all heard the saying that 75 percent of this game is played above the neck.

We want our training program to include the mental side as well as the physical. Getting the most from your workout means bringing more than just your muscles to the gym. To maximize our performance, we need our workout to be not only demanding and challenging but also efficient and precise. When you stay mentally locked and focused, you can put out 100 percent effort and get 100 percent of the benefit. When you lose focus, the effort could still be 100 percent, but the benefit is a far lower percentage. At these times we are apt to deviate from mechanics and perform the activity in a way that does more harm than good. Particularly when you are strength training, a raised level of focus is crucial. If necessary, work out with a partner and remind each other to keep your focus on correct technique.

CHAPTER 2

NUTRITION BASICS

As you know, when people search

the sports world for the best conditioned athletes, they barely even glance toward baseball. Take a look at some of the game's more visible players and you might understand why baseball players are not held up as prime examples of great conditioning. While football and hockey players need brute strength and speed, and basketball and soccer players require great stamina, baseball players seem to need only a great arm or a powerful swing. Because of baseball's long periods of what seems like low-intensity action, punctuated by great plays, casual observers might think that baseball players don't need to be fit to be good at the game. Of course, those of us closer to the game recognize such thinking as misguided.

In fact, complete conditioning, including sound nutrition, does help make baseball players better. Proper nutrition benefits players of all abilities and helps elevate the "natural athlete" to the next level. Despite the few exceptions you might be able to point out, the vast majority of baseball players simply cannot reach their full potential unless they eat right. Proper nutrition enables the body to make gains in size, strength, endurance, and conditioning. All the conditioning in the world will take you only part of the way toward improving your complete game. The other part depends on how well you fuel your body to perform the activity you require of it. Food deprivation and other improper diets jeopardize and limit the total strength and muscle-building process.

THE RIGHT MIX

Food fuels the body with energy. It seems only logical that someone exerting and expending more energy than another will require more fuel. But just *more* fuel is not enough. Just as a high-performance car requires a high-performance fuel, the highly trained athlete requires high-performance nutrients. These high-performance nutrients necessary for baseball players include the right mix of fluids, carbohydrates, proteins, and fats.

Fluids

Baseball players are often called the "boys of summer" because the game is played in the warm weather of summer. Warm weather climates mean that baseball players can lose more fluid through sweating than those who play cool-weather sports. When lost fluids are not replenished, the body's temperature rises, which usually causes faster exhaustion, a decrease in performance, and greater risk of heat injury. For these reasons, fluid intake is as necessary to the baseball player as a glove and a bat.

You avoid the risk of dehydration by replenishing your body regularly with fluids *prior* to the onset of thirst. If you wait until you're thirsty, you've waited too long. By drinking fluids, you also improve your performance by supplying your muscles with enough water for maximum muscle output. Not just any fluid will do. Cool water is best. Water between the temperatures of 40 and 50 degrees Fahrenheit will be absorbed faster by your intestines with less risk of cramping. The average person needs 64 ounces of water a day to maintain normal body functions. The well-trained baseball player needs at least that amount, and we recommend much more—at least 32 to 48 more ounces a day.

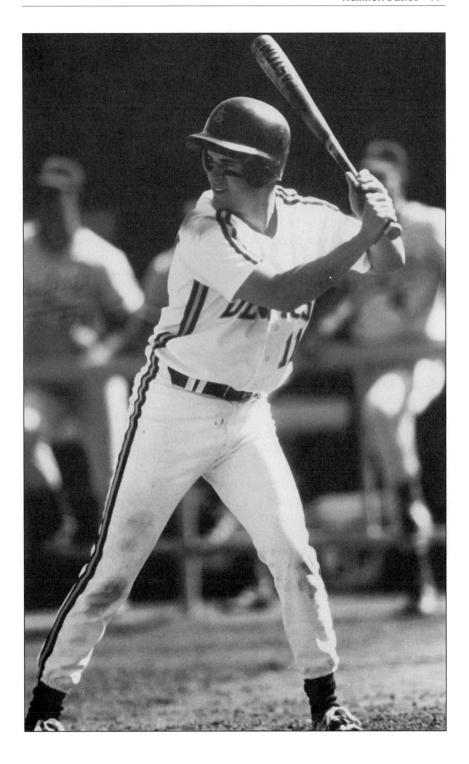

Consuming 12 to 14 eight-ounce glasses of water a day is a good practice to follow both in season and off season. Eating plenty of fruits and vegetables at meals and as snacks will also help replenish your fluids. As a bonus, these items are loaded with vital electrolytes, minerals, vitamins, and fiber—all necessary for your overall health.

Avoid fluids such as coffee, tea, and caffeinated soft drinks, as these do not rehydrate the body but act instead as diuretics, dehydrating you and robbing your body of precious nutrients. Also avoid alcohol, as it both dehydrates your body and inhibits performance. While sport drinks and juices provide water and are a good source of additional vitamins and carbohydrates, they tend to be more filling and can lead to less frequent intake. Again, water is the fluid of choice. For adequate hydration prior to a game or a workout, drink 2 1/2 cups of water two hours beforehand and another 1 1/2 cups 15 minutes before the practice or game begins. Remember—you'll need another 8 to 10 eight-ounce glasses a day on top of this.

Carbohydrates

Many consider carbohydrates the master fuel. For generating energy during practices and competition, they are definitely the fuel of choice. The body breaks carbohydrates down into glycogen, which directly supplies fuel to your muscles. The calories carbohydrates contain are also quickly and efficiently burned during exercise. Most researchers agree that athletes should keep their carbohydrate intake at 60 to 70 percent of their daily total calories.

There are two types of carbohydrates: complex and simple. Complex carbohydrates provide a gradual release of energy over a long period of time. Simple carbohydrates offer a quick but temporary rush of energy followed by low blood sugar, which can rob you of overall energy and performance intensity. Ideally, consume complex carbohydrates, which are found in fruits, root vegetables, beans, pasta, rice, grain breads, and cereals. Here are some foods that are high in carbohydrates:

Carbohydrates		
Breakfast	**Lunch/dinner**	**Dessert/snack**
Hot/cold cereal	Pasta with sauce	Angel food cake

Breakfast	Lunch/dinner	Dessert/snack
Pancakes/waffles	Vegetables	Pudding
Muffins	Bread/rolls	Oatmeal raisin
Toast/English muffin	Potato/rice/beans	cookies
Fruit/fruit juices	Fruit juices	Frozen yogurt
		Sherbet

Protein

When you hear the word *protein*, you used to think red meat. Today, the trend toward low-fat diets has shed light on the many other excellent sources of protein. And contrary to our old beliefs that athletes should consume great amounts of protein for muscle growth and repair, we now know that too much protein will only be converted to fat and can deter hydration. For an athlete, protein should account for 15 to 20 percent of the day's total calories.

Beef, pork, lamb, poultry, and fish are excellent animal sources of complete protein. Complete protein means that 90 to 95 percent of the protein is absorbed by the body. Try to eat only *lean* meats, not the cuts that are high in fat. Grains, nuts, beans, and tofu are also good sources of protein, but only about 75 percent of these nonanimal sources of protein are absorbed by the body. By limiting the amount of animal products consumed and including sources such as beans and dairy products in your diet, you should easily meet your daily protein requirement. Some complete protein foods include the following:

Complete Sources of Protein		
Meat	**Fish**	**Dairy**
Beef	Haddock	Cheese
Chicken	Salmon	Eggs
Ham	Tuna	Milk
Turkey		Yogurt

Fats

Despite all the bad press fat receives, it does have an important role in the athlete's diet as a source of concentrated energy. Although carbohydrate energy (glycogen) will be the first fuel your body uses during activity, you rely on energy from fat once the glycogen stores have been depleted. Glycogen is usually used up after about 30 minutes of strenuous activity. Because baseball rarely requires 30 minutes of straight activity, glycogen is the major fuel used in our game.

Ideally, limit your fat consumption to 15 to 20 percent of your total calories. Although fat does play a dietary role, too many fatty foods will likely lead to unnecessary and unwanted weight gain. Almost all foods contain some fat, but try to avoid high-fat sources such as fried foods, candy, potato chips, doughnuts, cookies, dairy products (whole milk, cheese, cream, butter, ice cream), mayonnaise, and red meats. There are several ways of lowering your fat intake without reducing taste or substance:

- Prepare foods by broiling, baking, steaming, or poaching rather than frying.
- Remove the skin from poultry and fish.
- Drink skim milk or water instead of whole milk.
- Substitute fish and white-meat chicken for red meats.
- Avoid foods packed in oil.

Again, you don't want to eliminate fat from your diet, but it's best to keep your intake below 20 percent of your daily calories.

PRE- AND POST-EVENT MEALS

Pre- and post-event nutrition is also very important. Whether training or playing, you should eat two to four hours before activity. This meal can prevent your blood sugar from getting too low, which can cause fatigue, dizziness, and other detrimental effects, and permits the absorption of carbohydrates as glycogen for optimal fuel use during exercise. Avoid overeating—eat only enough to fill your stomach to avoid hunger.

Before games, avoid foods with high cellulose content, such as lettuce, as they are more difficult to digest and can lead to gastrointestinal irritation. Avoid spicy and fatty fried foods for the same reason. Too

Nutritional Guidelines

When considering your dietary needs, remember the numbers for caloric intake:

Carbohydrates = 60 to 70 percent

Protein = 15 to 20 percent

Fat = 15 to 20 percent

Follow these general guidelines:

1. Eat breakfast. It is your foundation meal for the day—you should consume about one-third of your daily calories at breakfast.

2. Eat extra carbohydrates instead of extra protein.

3. Drink plenty of fluids, especially during hot weather.

4. Eat four to six small meals a day for better absorption of calories and nutrients.

5. Eat meals 2 to 4 hours before competition or training.

6. Eat within 1 to 1 1/2 hours after competition or training. Your body will absorb nutrients and replenish itself better at this time.

7. Don't eat late in the evening. Because you're relatively inactive at night, most calories won't be burned off and are instead stored as fat.

much protein and sugar intake can lead to dehydration and should be limited in pre-event meals. Liquids should be low in fat content and easily absorbed. Water is the best choice, but skim milk is also acceptable. Fruit juices can have a mild laxative effect, which might cause discomfort during activity. Don't drink beverages that contain caffeine because they act as diuretics and may increase pregame nervousness. Whether it be breakfast, lunch, or dinner, stick with a high-carbohydrate pre-event meal for optimal performance

Post-event nutrition is as important as pre-event nutrition. Eat your postgame or postpractice meal as soon after the game or practice as possible to replenish carbohydrates and other nutrients your body burned during activity. Ideally, you should eat no later than 60 to 90 minutes after the game, when your metabolism is at its highest. Your muscles are starving for nutritional replenishment, and at this time recuperating muscles will absorb the highest amount of nutrients from food. After 90 minutes, the body's metabolism begins to slow down and tends to store food as fat instead of converting it into energy for muscle stores.

It's also important to replenish your body's fluids soon after a game or practice. Fruit, fruit juices, and high-carbohydrate sport drinks are good sources for quick carbohydrate and nutrient replacement.

Late night postgame meals are common for baseball players. Keep in mind that your body will be slowing down because of the postgame recovery process and the time of day. Eat a high-carbohydrate, low-fat meal such as a turkey sub sandwich on wheat bread, or a grilled chicken or lean roast beef sandwich. Choose snacks low in fat such as unbuttered popcorn, fruits, raisins, bagels, pretzels, or graham crackers.

DINING OUT

When eating away from home—as more and more active people are doing to save time—you can still make healthy meal choices. In general, fast food is high in fat and low in such nutrients as calcium, vitamin C, and vitamin A, so you need to be careful when picking from the menu. Here are some suggestions from several popular fast-food restaurants:

Good Choices When Dining Out

Breakfast	Lunch/dinner
McDonald's Scrambled eggs English muffin with strawberry jam Orange juice	**McDonald's** Two chicken sandwiches Side salad with low-calorie dressing 2% milk
Wendy's Hot cakes with butter and syrup	**Wendy's** Two chicken breast sandwiches, no mayonnaise

Breakfast	Lunch/dinner

Wendy's
English muffin
  with strawberry jam
Orange juice
	Wendy's
	Baked potato or two servings
	  of chili
	2% milk

Arby's	**Arby's**
	Two junior roast beef
	  sandwiches with lettuce
	  and tomato
	2% milk

Taco Bell	**Taco Bell** Two tostados Two plain tortillas One bean burrito 2% milk
Pizza Hut	**Pizza Hut** Large spaghetti with meat sauce Breadsticks 2% milk or Medium cheese pizza Breadsticks 2% milk

STAYING AWAY FROM DRUGS, TOBACCO, AND ALCOHOL

As illogical as it seems, many high-profile athletes are lured by the glamour of their professions into using a variety of drugs, most notably alcohol and cocaine. Of course, these drugs do nothing to enhance performance on or off the playing field. Drugs lure athletes into a false sense of security, leading them to believe their game will improve—then the next they know they become dependent on the drug, both physically and psychologically. The addiction becomes consuming and soon robs the athlete of peak performance, and often also destroys his personal life. The best way to avoid this cycle is to simply not use any illegal drug such as cocaine, marijuana, steroids, or barbiturates. Even legal drugs such as tobacco, alcohol, and inhalants should be avoided, as they can be every bit as lethal as the illegal drugs.

Smokeless tobacco use by baseball players is widespread but has been aggressively attacked by the baseball community. It has been banned during competition in the minor leagues and at the high school level. Although smokeless tobacco remains allowed in the major leagues, many people in the baseball community, including ex–major leaguer Joe Garagiola, are actively lobbying to ban its use during competition at all levels of the game. Smokeless tobacco does pose serious health risks. Many people have died of oral or throat cancer caused by this habit. It can also lead to general periodontal destruction. But the substance contained in smokeless tobacco products, nitrosonornicotine, is more addictive than the nicotine found in cigarettes, so once you start chewing, it can be hard to quit. As with all other drug use, it's best not to start at all.

CHAPTER 3

FLEXIBILITY AND WARM-UP

Before beginning a workout or any other physical activity, you need to warm up your muscles and stretch. Although many people think that stretching is a part of the warm-up, the two activities are actually different parts of your program. You should warm up your muscles before you stretch them. Warming up raises the temperature of your deep muscles and connective tissues, allowing for greater flexibility, reducing the possibility of muscle tears and ligament strains, and helping prevent muscle soreness. Stretching focuses on increasing flexibility, which is the range of movement of a joint or joint group as influenced by the surrounding muscle and connective tissues. A good stretching routine aids in decreasing joint injuries, and greater flexibility contributes to improved athletic performance.

WARMING UP

A proper warm-up, though key to any training program, is often underrated or ignored by many coaches and players. Stretching is not a replacement for warming up the body in preparation for training. Our purpose in warming up is to prepare the body through gradual movements for the full effort it will perform following the warm-up. Three goals to warming up include

1. creating internal muscular warmth and through slow stretching movements preparing nerves and joints for the explosive movements to come,

2. implementing biomechanically correct movements that incorporate fast fire actions at a low intensity, and

3. gaining full range of motion with dynamic and static stretches *after* muscles have become warm and flexible.

As noted, a chief objective in warming up is to prepare your muscles, tendons, and ligaments for the explosiveness of strength and speed training. It is more important to warm the body up through gradual movements and acceleration than slow stretching alone. Properly warmed muscles respond much more quickly to neural stimuli than unwarmed muscles do—this is important in preventing injury.

Your warm-up can be a variety of several exercises. What we call a continuous warm-up includes performing a combination of the technical skills involved in your sport or activity. This warm-up routine gradually warms the muscles while teaching proper and new neuromuscular patterns. A good warm-up consists of 10 to 15 minutes of continuous exercise. Varying your warm-up will make it more enjoyable and upbeat. We list several warm-up exercises at the end of the chapter, but here are some other suggestions:

1. Jog slowly 20 to 30 yards back and forth, four to six times, keeping the distance and time constant.

2. Jog while doing arm circles on either side.

3. Jog while raising your arms overhead and back down to your sides.

4. Combine high knees (exaggerated skipping) with large arm swings.

6. Side-shuffle 20 to 30 yards; change sides and return.

7. Back pedal 20 to 30 yards back and forth several times.

8. Perform cariocas, side-shuffling while crossing one foot over and then behind the other (left over right, step right, left behind right, step right, and repeat). Return facing the same direction but starting with the other foot.

You can perform all these movements and skills while playing tag or relay games. Or you can make the warm-up competitive by running partner or team relays and backward and forward races. The main objective is to warm up the muscles, and since there are dozens of ways of doing this, there's no excuse for letting your routine become stale.

STRETCHING

Flexibility and stretching have always been a part of baseball. It used to be that the warm-up routine consisted mainly of stretching exercises. Now we understand that warming the muscles is probably more important than stretching them. Although many people still believe that poor flexibility increases your chances of getting hurt, in fact this condition has never been proven to be the primary cause of an injury. If you pull a quadriceps muscle, it's not just because you lack flexibility. However, a lack of flexibility *can* hinder performance. If you are tight through your hamstrings and lower back, your running mechanics will be affected. When poor flexibility starts to limit your performance, you need to increase your range of motion through a good stretching program.

There are four basics types of stretching techniques, including static stretching, dynamic or ballistic stretching, slow movement stretching, and PNF stretching.

Static Stretching

Static stretching, the most common stretching technique, consists of a voluntary passive relaxation of the elongated muscle. The main advantage of static stretching is that you can do it without assistance. In a static stretch, you slowly and gently stretch a muscle to the point of tension, causing a slight discomfort that should never reach the point of pain. At the point the stretch becomes uncomfortable, hold it for 10 to 15 seconds, then repeat the stretch on the opposite side.

Dynamic or Ballistic Stretching

Ballistic stretching places the joint and muscle group in a stretched position and then bounces slightly against the stretch. Some frown upon this method because of its rapid contraction of the muscle, but the advantage to dynamic stretching is that it prepares the range of motion for a larger joint and muscle group. These stretches closely resemble the ballistic movements required in baseball, such as running, throwing, and hitting. To some degree, with proper technique and instruction, you should incorporate dynamic stretching into your stretching routine. Keep in mind, however, that if performed too aggressively or when muscles are not properly warmed, this type of stretching can cause muscle tears or pulls. It is extremely important to perform these stretches in a controlled manner in order to avoid muscle damage.

Slow Movement Stretching

The value of slow movement stretches are that they serve as a form of warm-up. Slow movement stretches such as neck rotations, arm rotation, and trunk rotation help to slowly stretch and warm muscles. The movements are similar to dynamic stretches but are not as violent on the muscle while allowing for the same flexibility gains.

Proprioceptive Neuromuscular Facilitation (PNF)

PNF stretching is a good option for the athlete who is very tight and wants to aggressively increase flexibility. This kind of stretching requires a workout partner and takes more time than the other stretches. The partner holds you in a stretched position while you contract the muscle and push against your partner's resistance. This method is used in rehabilitation and also to stretch a pitcher's shoulder area. PNF stretching is one of the best methods for increasing ranges of motion— but it is also potentially dangerous if performed improperly or without good concentration from your partner, who must apply resistance slowly and smoothly.

Which Stretch Is Best?

Which stretching technique you employ depends on your knowledge of the stretch and the effectiveness of the technique as it applies to your sport. Baseball players use static stretching as the primary stretch because of its tradition and because it can be done without assistance. However, to maximize a stretching program, all four methods should be incorporated to some extent. All stretches are effective, but because of the risk involved in PNF stretches, we recommend using static and slow movement stretches primarily, as these can be performed individually and the intensity levels can be controlled. Combining slow movement and static stretching will help increase your range of motion and also prepare you for upcoming movement and exercises.

COOLING DOWN

An active cooldown after exercising is recommended to decrease lactic acid levels in the blood and muscles. By gradually diminishing the work intensity, you keep the muscle pumps active while preventing blood from pooling in your arms and legs. Jogging for 30 to 60 seconds followed by three to five minutes of walking is usually sufficient for circulation and various body functions to return to pre-exercise levels. A light static stretch is also advised after a workout to help circulate the lactic acid in the muscles and prevent muscle soreness.

HIGH-KNEE SKIPS

Focus: To elevate body temperature and warm and stretch hamstrings, gluteals, and quadriceps area

Procedure:

1.   In a skipping motion, lift your knees toward your shoulders.
2.   Follow proper running form, pulling toe up, heel up, and knee up.
3.   Work your arms to get foot-arm action. Opposite arm, opposite leg.

Distance: 10 to 15 yards, repeating two to three times.

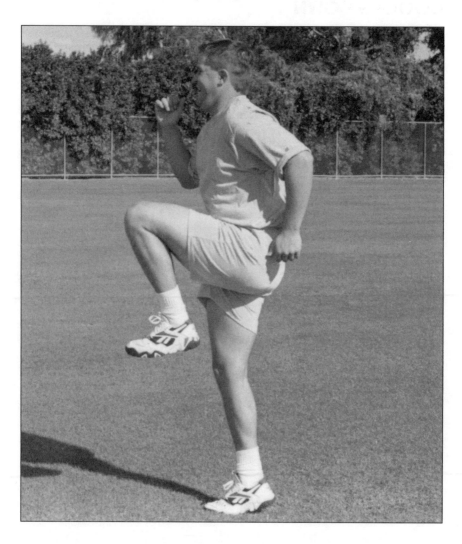

BUTT KICKS

Focus: To warm hamstrings and gluteals and practice proper running form

Procedure:

1. Staying on the balls of your feet, try to touch your butt with your heels.
2. Do not lift your knee. Point the knee straight toward the ground during the exercise.
3. Move your legs in a fast and aggressive but controlled pace.

Distance: 10 to 15 yards

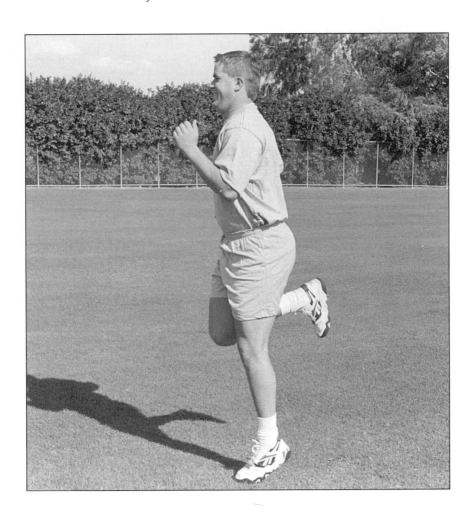

ARM KICKS

Focus: To warm hamstrings and gluteals

Procedure:

1. With a skip, extend a straight left leg up to your left arm, then repeat with the opposite leg and arm.

2. Perform this drill slowly, with control.

3. Excellent warm-up exercise also teaches the aggressive firing pattern of the gluteals and hamstrings and the driving action of the feet when you sprint.

Distance: 10 yards

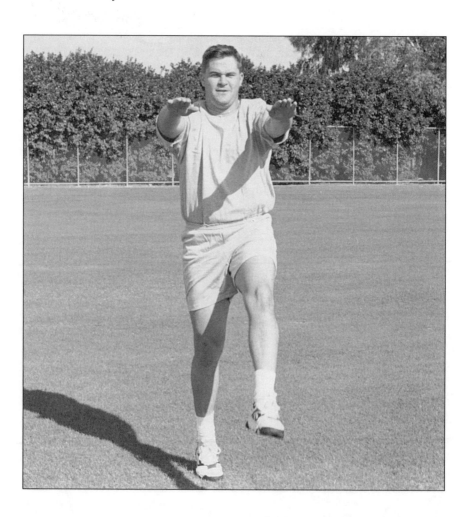

OUT AND OVER KICKS

Focus: To warm up and increase range of motion in the groin and inner thighs

Procedure:

1. With a skip or light run, kick your leg out and over in a large circular motion, then repeat with other leg.

2. Perform this exercise with control.

Distance: 10 yards

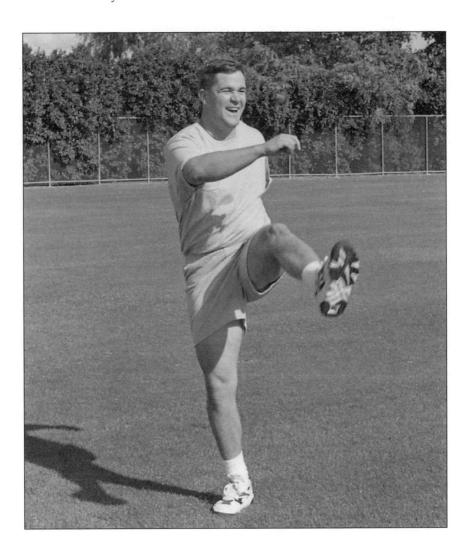

KNEE-TO-SHOULDER LIFTS

Focus: To warm hip flexors, hamstrings, and gluteals

Procedure:

1. While skipping, lock your hands and place them in front of your chest or belly.

2. Using good leg lift mechanics, try to drive your right knee up to your right shoulder.

3. Repeat with other leg.

Distance: 10 to 15 yards

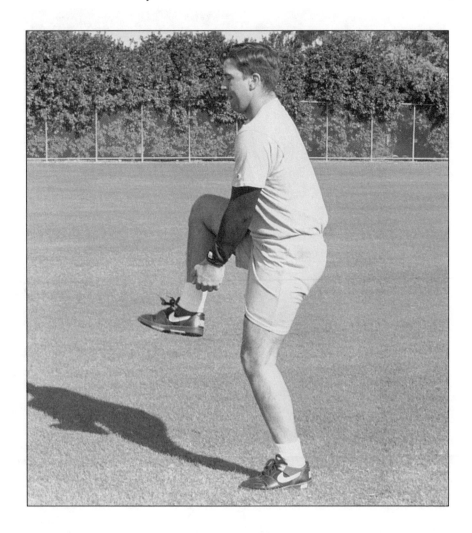

Note: All of the following static stretches can be performed with a partner's assistance to create PNF stretches. However, we don't recommend PNF stretching except under strict supervision by a professional.

NECK STRETCHES

Focus: Neck and trapezius muscles

Procedure:

1. Stand with feet shoulder-width apart and knees slightly flexed.

2. Place both hands under your chin and gently push your chin up until the back of your head rests on your shoulders.

3. Hold this stretch for 10 to 20 seconds.

4. Take your right hand across the top of your head and rest your hand on your left ear.

Duration: Repeat the stretch on opposite side.

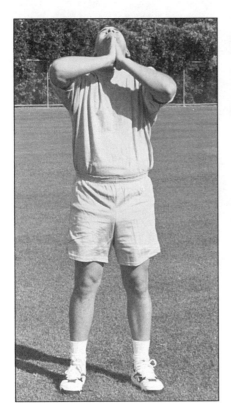 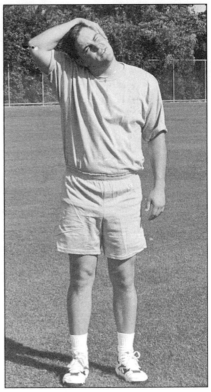

STANDING SPINAL TWIST

Focus: Lower and upper back

Procedure:

1.   Stand with your feet together, legs straight, and hands on each hip.
2.   Keeping your torso upright, turn and slowly twist to your left to look at your left heel.
3.   Hold this stretch for 10 to 20 seconds and then repeat to opposite side.

Duration: Repeat on opposite side one time.

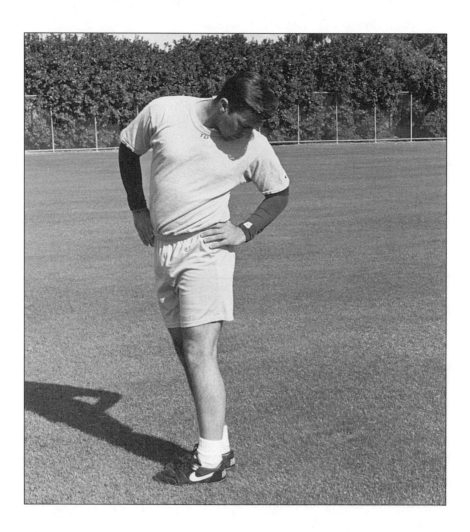

TRICEPS SHOULDER STRETCH

Focus: Triceps and rear deltoid area

Procedure:

1. Stand with your feet shoulder-width apart and knees slightly bent.
2. Place your right hand behind your head with your elbow bent and your palm flat in the middle of your back.
3. With your opposite hand, gently apply pressure to your right elbow.
4. Repeat on the opposite side.

Duration: Hold stretch 10 to 20 seconds each side one time.

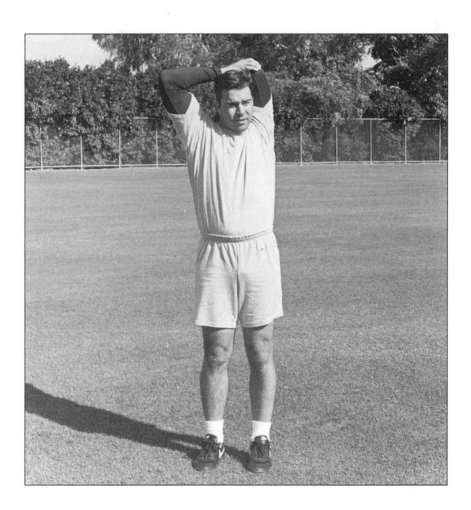

FOREARM AND WRIST STRETCH

Focus: Muscles of the lower arm

Procedure:

1. With your left arm extended in front of your body and parallel to the ground, point your left hand and fingers toward the sky.

2. Place your right hand at the base of the fingers of your left hand and gently pull back toward your body.

3. Hold the stretch for 10 to 15 seconds.

4. Pointing your fingers toward the ground, gently pull back toward your body with your right hand and hold for 10 to 15 seconds.

Duration: Repeat on opposite side one time.

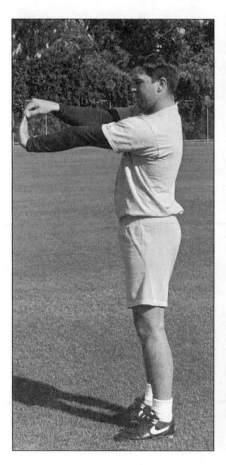 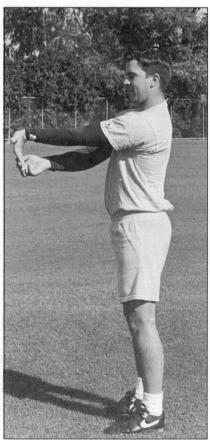

LUNGE

Focus: Hip flexors, quadriceps, groin

Procedure:

1. In a lunge position, extend your left leg out in front while keeping your heel flat.
2. Extend your right leg back and right foot up on your toes.
3. With your left knee bent at about a 45-degree angle, lower your right knee about five inches from the ground.
4. Place hand on your left quadriceps area. To increase the stretch, lower your chest toward your thighs.

Duration: Hold stretch 10 to 20 seconds each leg one time.

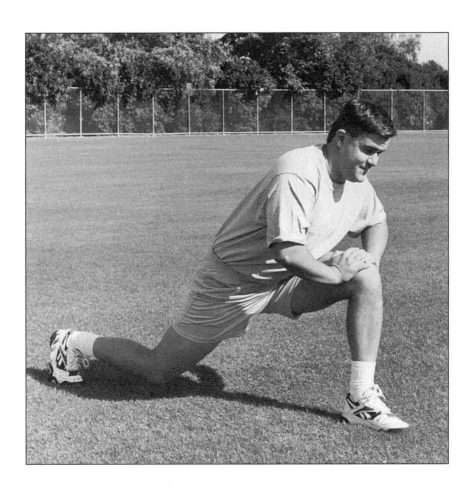

SIDE HURDLE STRETCH

Focus: Groin, gluteals, hamstrings, hip flexors

Procedure:

1. Start standing with your legs spread at arms' width and both feet facing forward.

2. Bend to the right and lower your butt down until your right thigh is parallel to the ground. Keep your right heel as flat as possible and your torso upright.

3. Your left leg is extended to the side, straight and with your foot facing forward and flat.

4. For a variation, turn your foot on its heel with your toes pointing up to focus more on the hamstrings.

Duration: Hold stretch 10 to 20 seconds for each leg one time.

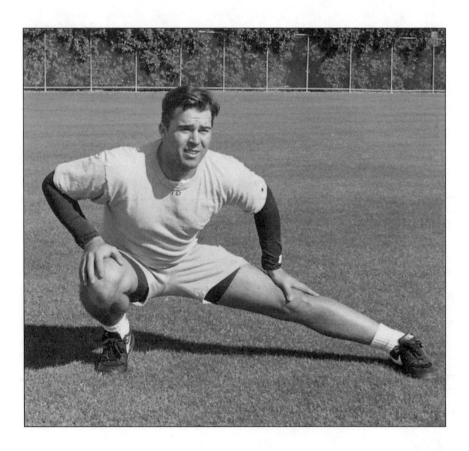

SITTING V STRETCH

Focus: Hamstrings, gluteals, lower back

Procedure:

1. In a seated upright position, spread your legs wide in a V shape, keeping them as straight as possible.

2. Slowly lower your chest toward your right thigh. Extend your right hand out toward your right toe.

3. Grab your toe and hold this position.

4. Use your left hand to help increase the stretch by pressing down on your right knee to keep your leg straight or by extending it to grab your left foot.

Duration: Hold 10 to 20 seconds each side one time.

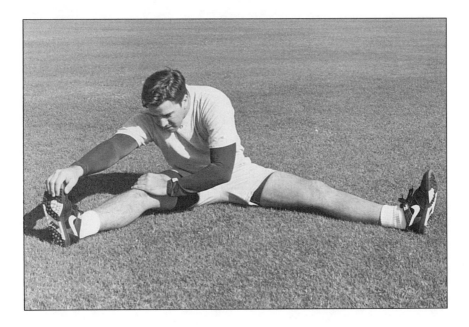

BUTTERFLY STRETCH

Focus: Groin, inner thigh

Procedure:

1. In a seated and tall upright position, bring your feet together between your legs and grab your feet or ankles.

2. Relax your groin area and force your knees toward the ground.

3. To increase the intensity, use your elbow to lightly apply downward pressure on your knees.

Duration: Hold the stretch 10 to 20 seconds one time.

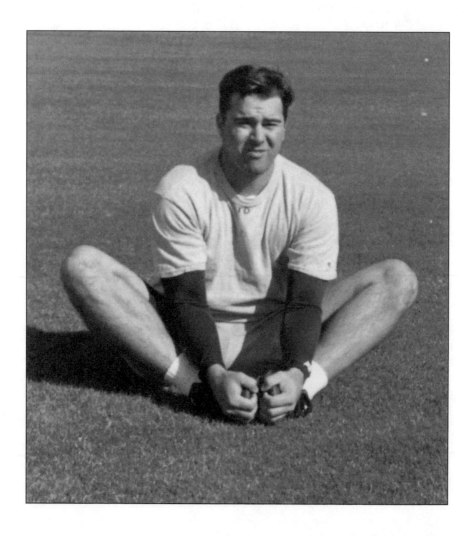

SEATED SPINAL TWIST

Focus: Lower back, outside gluteals

Procedure:

1. In a seated upright position, cross your bent left leg across your straight right leg.
2. Twist your trunk and lower your back to the left.
3. Take your right arm across your body and place your elbow on the outside of your left knee.
4. Apply force with your right elbow as you twist your upper torso around.

Duration: 10 to 20 seconds on each side one time.

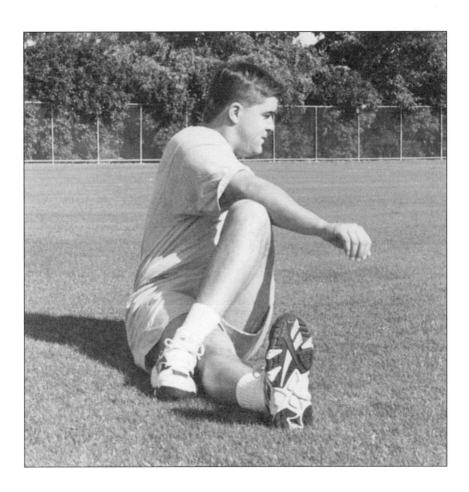

CHAPTER 4

STRENGTH TRAINING

The game of baseball requires you

to use all of the major muscle groups of your body. Throwing, catching, hitting, and running demand the power of the leg muscles, the hip flexors and gluteals, the support of the abdominal and back muscles, and the skill and strength of the shoulder, chest, and arm muscles. While some sports require higher levels of strength, all baseball activities require a certain degree of strength. We want to build strength primarily in our core area to help increase our speed and power, not to bulk up or build mass. Bulking up can actually hamper the execution of baseball skills. Rather, to optimize baseball skills through strength training, you'll want to focus on sport-specific strength gains.

With all the information out there on weight programs, it can be hard to decipher what's good and bad for players. Coaches should be responsible for gathering strength-training information specific to baseball and creating a program based on that information. Briefly, here are the basic goals of a properly administered weight program:

1. To increase muscle strength and endurance
2. To increase flexibility and range of motion
3. To strengthen connective tissue (tendons, ligaments, overall joint stability
4. To improve neuromuscular (muscle and nerve) efficiency
5. To decrease chance of injury
6. To shorten rehabilitation time in the event of injury
7. To aid in player longevity

BUILDING A STRENGTH FOUNDATION

Strength training is one of our foundations for building a better athlete. It serves as a strong base for any effective training program. All the speed, agility, and baseball drills in the world will do little to enhance your game if you don't have the necessary strength to perform them correctly and effectively. To use the example given in chapter 1: To increase speed, more power must be exerted against the ground; to exert more power requires greater strength. Often it's not an athlete's lack of ability, will, or effort that limits his performance but a lack of physical strength. This is why strength training becomes such an important part of your complete conditioning routine.

When designing your strength program, focus the majority of your training during the off-season. During the season, you don't want to tax your muscles and cause added fatigue through a vigorous weight-training program. Instead, incorporate an active strength program in which players weight train three times a week throughout the off-season. The program should peak during the preseason, when workouts should be done two to three times a week. Once the season begins, limit your workouts to one to two times a week. Remember that key factors in any sound strength-training program are intensity and the overload principle. If you don't incorporate these principles into your program, your strength gains will be minimized.

INTENSITY

In chapter 1 we defined intensity as the power output (rate of performing work) of an exercise. Intensity in lifting weights can be increased by adding weight or moving a given resistance faster. High achievers are willing to work hard. The intensity of an exercise must challenge your athletes. When prepared and organized properly, intense efforts do not drain the athlete but vitalize him and move him closer to his goal. Great players like Nolan Ryan, Will Clark, Dennis Eckersly, and many others are fierce competitors whose intensity levels are very high. They are extremely focused when they're on the field, and it shows in their ability to perform at exceptional levels. Every athlete wants to feel self-worth—the effort to achieve this goal and become a better player should be worth giving.

But intensity is relative. What's intense for one person may be easy for another. In strength training, we know intensity is the tension of stress put on the muscle, and we know people have varying intensity levels. So, how do we measure intensity? By using a percentage of a player's one repetition maximum (1RM). The 1RM can be an estimation of the person's maximum lift if a maximum test cannot be performed. If we want athletes to work in different intensity zones, we define those areas this way:

Heavy: 90 to 100 percent or more

Medium: 70 to 90 percent

Light: 0 to 70 percent

Example: A player has a 1RM of 200 pounds in the bench press. If his workout calls for 80 percent of 200 pounds, he will work out at 160 pounds for that day.

When these variables are manipulated, athletes make faster gains. For instance, it is not recommended to handle maximum poundage at every workout session or to work at the same intensity at each workout. Effective increase in training stress through variation of intensity is a good practice to keep the muscle from becoming stagnant.

The maximum lift chart (table 4.1) helps athletes figure out the percentage of 1RM they need to work at on given workouts. Example: If an athlete's maximum leg press is 250 pounds, you simply look up 250 pounds on the maximum lift chart. If you want the athlete to work at 65 percent of his maximum for a prescribed number of reps, scroll over to 65 percent down to the 250-pound line and you find that 65 percent of 250 pounds is 160 pounds.

Table 4.1 Maximum Lift Chart

Number of repetitions

	1	2	3	4	5	6	7	8	9	10	11	12								
Lb.	97%	95%	92%	90%	87%	85%	82%	80%	77%	75%	72%	70%	67%	65%	62%	60%	57%	55%	52%	50%
70	65	65	65	65	60	60	60	55	55	50	50	50	45	45	45	50	40	40	35	35
80	75	75	75	70	70	70	65	65	65	60	60	55	55	55	50	50	45	45	45	40
90	85	85	85	80	80	75	75	70	70	70	65	65	60	60	55	55	50	50	45	45
100	95	95	95	90	90	85	85	80	80	75	70	70	70	65	65	60	60	55	55	50
110	105	105	100	100	95	95	90	90	85	80	80	80	75	70	70	65	65	60	60	55
120	115	115	110	110	105	100	100	95	90	90	85	85	80	80	75	70	70	65	65	60
130	125	125	120	115	115	110	105	105	100	100	95	90	90	85	80	80	75	70	70	65
140	135	135	130	125	125	120	115	110	110	105	100	100	95	90	90	85	80	75	75	70
150	145	145	140	135	130	130	125	120	115	110	110	105	100	100	95	90	85	85	80	75
160	150	150	145	145	140	135	130	130	125	120	115	110	110	105	100	95	95	90	85	80
170	165	160	155	155	150	145	140	135	130	125	120	120	115	110	105	100	100	95	90	85
180	175	170	165	160	155	155	150	145	140	135	130	125	120	115	115	110	105	100	95	90
190	185	180	175	170	165	160	155	150	150	145	140	135	130	125	120	115	110	105	100	95
200	195	190	185	180	175	170	165	160	155	150	145	140	135	130	125	120	115	110	105	100
210	205	200	195	190	185	180	175	170	160	155	150	145	140	135	130	125	120	115	110	105
220	215	210	205	200	195	185	180	175	170	165	160	155	150	145	140	130	125	120	115	110
230	225	220	210	210	200	195	190	185	175	170	165	160	155	150	145	140	130	125	120	115
240	235	230	220	215	210	205	200	190	185	180	170	170	160	155	150	145	140	130	125	120
250	245	240	230	225	220	210	205	200	190	185	180	175	170	160	155	150	145	140	130	125
260	255	245	240	235	230	220	215	210	200	195	185	180	175	170	160	155	150	145	135	130

(continued)

Table 4.1   Maximum Lift Chart

Number of repetitions

										12	11	10	9	8	7	6	5	4	3	2	1
Lb.	50%	52%	55%	57%	60%	62%	65%	67%	70%	72%	75%	77%	80%	82%	85%	87%	90%	92%	95%	97%
270	135	140	150	155	160	170	175	180	190	195	200	205	215	225	230	235	245	250	255	265
280	140	145	155	160	170	175	180	190	195	200	210	215	225	230	240	245	250	260	265	275
290	145	150	160	165	175	180	190	195	205	210	215	225	230	240	245	255	260	270	275	285
300	150	160	165	180	180	190	195	200	210	215	225	230	240	250	255	265	270	280	285	295
310	155	165	170	180	185	195	200	210	215	225	230	240	250	255	265	270	280	285	295	300
320	160	170	175	185	190	200	210	215	225	230	240	245	255	265	270	280	290	295	305	310
330	165	175	180	185	200	205	215	220	230	235	245	255	265	270	280	290	295	305	315	320
340	170	180	185	195	205	215	220	230	240	245	255	260	270	280	290	300	305	315	325	330
350	175	185	190	200	210	220	230	235	245	255	260	270	280	290	300	305	315	325	330	340
360	180	190	200	205	215	225	235	245	250	260	270	280	290	295	305	315	325	335	340	350
370	185	195	205	215	220	230	240	250	260	270	280	285	295	305	315	325	330	340	350	360
380	190	200	210	220	230	240	245	255	265	275	285	295	305	315	325	335	340	350	360	370
390	195	205	215	225	235	245	255	265	275	285	295	300	310	320	330	340	350	360	370	380
400	200	210	220	230	240	250	260	270	280	290	300	310	320	330	340	350	360	370	380	390
410	205	215	225	235	245	255	265	275	285	295	310	320	330	340	350	360	370	380	390	400
420	210	220	230	240	250	265	275	285	295	305	315	325	335	345	360	370	380	390	400	410
430	215	225	235	245	260	270	280	290	300	310	320	335	345	355	365	375	390	400	410	420
440	220	230	240	255	265	275	285	295	310	320	330	340	350	365	375	385	395	405	420	430
450	225	235	250	260	270	280	290	305	315	325	340	350	360	370	380	395	405	415	430	440

(continued)

Table 4.1 Maximum Lift Chart

Number of repetitions

| | | | | | | | | | | 12 | 11 | 10 | 9 | 8 | 7 | 6 | 5 | 4 | 3 | 2 | 1 |
Lb.	50%	52%	55%	57%	60%	62%	65%	67%	70%	72%	75%	77%	80%	82%	85%	87%	90%	92%	95%	97%
460	230	240	255	265	275	290	300	310	320	335	345	355	370	380	390	405	415	425	440	450
470	235	245	260	270	280	295	305	320	330	340	350	365	375	390	400	410	425	435	445	460
480	240	250	265	275	290	300	310	325	335	350	360	370	385	395	410	420	430	445	455	470
490	245	255	270	280	295	305	320	330	345	355	370	380	390	405	415	430	440	455	465	480
500	250	260	275	285	300	315	325	340	350	365	375	390	400	415	425	440	450	465	475	490
510	255	265	280	295	305	320	330	345	360	370	385	395	410	420	435	445	460	470	485	495
520	260	275	285	300	310	325	340	350	365	375	390	405	415	430	440	455	470	480	495	505
530	265	280	290	305	320	330	345	360	370	385	400	410	425	435	450	465	475	490	505	515
540	270	285	295	310	325	335	350	365	380	390	405	420	430	445	460	475	485	500	515	525
550	275	290	300	315	330	345	360	370	385	400	410	425	440	455	470	480	495	510	520	535
560	280	295	310	320	335	350	365	380	390	405	420	435	450	460	475	490	500	515	530	545
570	285	300	315	330	340	355	370	385	400	415	430	440	455	470	485	500	515	525	540	555
580	290	305	320	335	350	360	375	390	405	420	435	450	465	480	490	505	520	535	550	565
590	295	310	325	340	355	370	385	400	415	430	440	455	470	485	500	515	530	545	560	575
600	300	315	330	345	360	375	390	405	420	435	450	465	480	495	510	525	540	555	570	585
610	305	320	335	350	365	380	395	410	425	440	460	475	490	505	520	535	550	565	580	595
620	310	315	340	355	370	390	405	420	435	450	465	480	495	510	530	545	560	575	590	605
630	315	330	345	360	380	395	410	425	440	455	470	490	505	520	535	550	570	585	600	615
640	320	335	350	370	385	400	415	430	450	465	480	495	510	530	545	560	575	590	610	625
650	325	340	355	375	390	405	420	440	455	470	485	505	520	535	550	570	585	600	615	635

(continued)

Table 4.1   Maximum Lift Chart

Number of repetitions

									12	11	10	9	8	7	6	5	4	3	2	1
Lb.	50%	52%	55%	57%	60%	62%	65%	67%	70%	72%	75%	77%	80%	82%	85%	87%	90%	92%	95%	97%
660	330	345	360	380	395	415	430	445	460	480	495	510	530	545	560	580	595	610	625	645
670	335	350	370	385	400	420	435	450	470	485	500	520	535	555	570	585	605	620	635	655
680	340	355	375	390	410	425	440	460	475	495	510	525	545	560	580	595	610	630	645	665
690	345	360	380	395	415	430	450	465	485	500	515	535	550	570	585	605	620	640	655	675
700	350	365	385	400	420	435	455	470	490	505	525	540	560	580	595	615	630	650	665	685
710	355	370	390	410	425	445	460	480	495	515	530	550	570	585	605	620	640	655	675	690
720	360	375	395	410	430	450	470	485	505	520	540	560	575	595	610	630	650	665	685	700
730	365	380	400	420	440	455	475	490	510	530	550	565	585	600	620	640	655	675	695	710
740	370	385	405	425	445	465	480	500	520	535	555	575	590	610	630	650	665	685	700	720
750	375	395	415	430	450	470	490	505	525	545	560	580	600	620	640	655	675	695	710	730
760	380	395	420	435	455	470	495	510	530	545	565	585	610	625	645	660	685	700	720	735
770	385	400	425	440	460	475	500	515	540	555	580	595	615	630	655	670	695	710	730	745
780	390	405	430	445	470	485	505	525	545	560	585	600	625	640	665	680	700	720	740	755
790	395	410	435	450	475	490	515	530	555	570	595	610	630	650	670	690	710	725	750	765
800	400	415	440	455	480	495	520	535	560	575	600	615	640	655	680	695	720	735	760	775
810	405	420	445	460	485	500	525	540	565	585	610	625	650	665	690	705	730	745	770	785
820	410	425	450	465	490	510	535	550	575	590	615	630	655	670	700	715	740	755	780	795
830	415	430	455	475	500	515	540	555	580	600	625	640	665	680	705	720	750	765	790	805
840	420	435	460	480	505	520	545	565	590	605	630	645	670	690	715	730	755	775	800	815

(continued)

Table 4.1 Maximum Lift Chart (continued)

Number of repetitions

Lb.	50%	52%	55%	57%	60%	62%	65%	67%	12 70%	11 72%	10 75%	9 77%	8 80%	7 82%	6 85%	5 87%	4 90%	3 92%	2 95%	1 97%
850	425	440	470	485	510	525	555	570	595	610	640	655	680	695	725	740	765	780	810	825
860	430	445	475	490	515	535	560	575	600	620	645	660	690	705	730	750	775	790	815	835
870	435	450	480	495	520	540	565	585	610	625	655	670	695	715	740	755	785	800	825	845
880	440	460	485	500	530	545	570	590	615	635	660	680	705	720	750	765	790	810	835	855
890	445	465	490	505	535	550	580	595	625	640	670	685	710	730	755	775	800	820	845	865
900	450	470	495	515	540	560	585	605	630	650	675	695	720	740	765	785	810	830	855	875
910	455	475	500	520	545	565	590	610	635	655	685	700	730	745	775	790	820	835	865	885
920	460	480	505	525	550	570	600	615	645	660	690	710	735	755	780	800	830	845	875	890
930	465	485	510	530	560	575	605	625	650	670	695	715	745	765	790	810	835	855	885	900
940	470	490	515	535	565	585	610	630	660	675	705	725	750	770	800	820	845	865	895	910
950	475	495	520	540	570	590	620	635	665	685	715	730	760	780	810	825	855	875	905	920
960	480	500	530	545	575	595	625	645	670	690	720	740	770	785	815	835	865	885	910	930
970	485	505	535	555	580	600	630	650	680	700	730	745	775	795	825	845	875	890	920	940
980	490	510	540	560	590	610	635	655	685	705	735	755	785	805	835	855	880	900	930	950
990	495	515	545	565	595	615	645	665	695	715	745	760	790	810	840	860	890	910	940	960
1000	500	520	550	570	600	620	650	670	700	720	750	770	800	820	850	870	900	920	950	970
1010	505	525	555	575	605	625	655	675	705	725	760	780	810	830	860	880	910	930	960	980
1020	510	530	560	580	610	630	665	685	715	735	765	785	815	835	870	890	920	940	970	990
1030	515	535	565	585	615	635	670	690	720	740	770	790	820	840	875	895	925	945	975	995
1040	520	540	570	595	625	645	675	695	730	750	780	800	830	855	885	905	935	955	990	1010

THE OVERLOAD PRINCIPLE

For a muscle to get stronger, it must be overloaded. The overload principle simply means putting stress (amount of weight) on the muscle greater than what it is used to. The game of baseball demands great devotion of physical energies. Great players like Barry Larkin, Paul Molitor, and Ozzie Smith view these mental and physical demands as challenges, not as boring chores. The love and passion required to play this game needs to be reflected in your preparation. For improvement to occur in your workouts, you must impose a demand on the body system. Studies have shown that baseball players should train at loads between 70 and 90 percent of their maximum for strength and speed to be optimally increased. Loads greater than 90 percent produce no additional measurable strength and lead to shortened workouts due to early "maxing out" or tiring. Anything less than 70 percent leads to the increase in mass that athletes such as body builders and football players work to achieve. These percentages should not be confused with cardio-vascular exercise targets, which target heart rates.

Most of us are familiar with the immediate results associated with a new program. Right from the start, your muscles feel firmer and stronger. The motivation and the discipline are there, and the results come quickly. But as the weeks pass, the progress starts to slow down. The same workout that was once so motivating becomes boring. You don't have the same zip or pep as in the beginning. Well, that same feeling also applies to muscles after they repeat the same work day after day—they get "bored," and their progress slows. As an analogy of this process, think that every time you lift, you're breaking down muscle fibers. These fibers are basic building blocks of the muscle. The rebuilding of these fibers is what adds mass to the muscle and makes you stronger. However, the body being the finely tuned, intricate machine it is will use only the amount of muscle fibers necessary to complete the job. Studies have shown that the body can adapt to new exercise routines in as few as three or four workouts. Consequently, you need to constantly shock your muscles with something they haven't done before. Adaptation and exercise change will be discussed in chapter 11, Training Programs.

FULL RANGE OF MOTION AND LIFTING MECHANICS

Wasted productivity is probably one of the biggest villains in the weight room. I think we're all guilty of it—the swinging of weights or exhibiting bad mechanics when we try to lift too much weight. Baseball places tremendous stress on joints and ligaments. Strong emphasis is on throwing mechanics to help protect the shoulder girdle and elbow to minimize this stress. So why would we want to go to the weight room and defeat this whole protection process by lifting improperly?

In order to make them stronger and to take some stress off the tendons and ligaments, muscles must be worked through a full range of motion. Muscle contractions occur quite rapidly when the muscle is doing work. But if we start to increase intensity without control or start moving the weight faster than the muscle can contract, serious amounts of undue stress are placed on joint areas. When momentum gets the better of the athlete in the weight room, the joints rather than the muscle end up taking the stress to try to control or stop the weight. This can easily cause an injury.

Proper lifting mechanics lead to muscles being worked through a full range of motion. A muscle that is strong through its full range is more explosive and can generate more reactive power. Improper posterior alignment such as hanging your head, hunching your shoulders, or swaying your back shortens the spine and limits the range of motion in joints and muscles. This places undue stress on ligaments, tendons, and the lower back and again increases your risk of injury. Ballistic and uncontrolled movements often associated with too heavy weights, poor mechanics, and improperly prepared programs are not beneficial for or conducive to becoming better baseball players.

If you've spent much time in weight rooms, you've seen those athletes who approach weight training with lots of enthusiasm and brawn but not much brain. We call them "danger rangers" because they are prime candidates for a weightlifting injury caused by unskilled technique. Don't you be a danger ranger—give lifting the care and control it deserves.

CORE AREA

The abdominal muscles, back muscles, gluteals, hips, and chest and shoulder muscles make up what we call the core area of the body. The core is the main target area for athletic performance. These areas must be well conditioned and strong for optimal performance. The primary function of the core is to transfer force generated by the lower body to the chest, shoulders, and arms, where the force is applied. The action and strength of this core area contributes to over 50 percent of the force generated in throwing and hitting. This area also stabilizes the trunk area when running. Because of its great importance in baseball, we'll say quite a bit about strengthening the core area. First, let's focus on the core areas and core exercises that apply in the weight room.

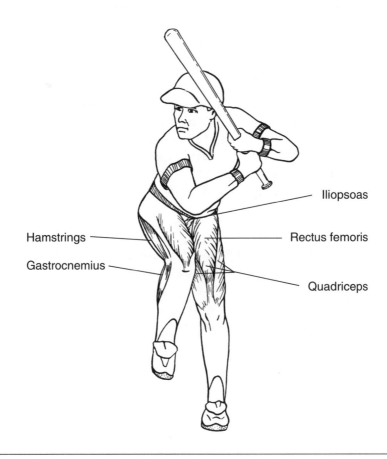

Major leg and hip muscles.

LEGS AND HIP REGION

The legs and hip region is undoubtedly the most important area for any athlete involved in a movement sport. This region contains some of the largest and strongest muscles in the body, including the muscle groups at the front and back part of the legs known as quadriceps and hamstrings. These groups drive the muscles of the gluteals area and hip flexors, which serve like firing pistons in explosive movements such as running and jumping. Development of these large muscle groups in the body's power zone is best achieved through specific core exercises.

SQUAT

Unique and unparalleled in its position of eminence in athletic strength training and conditioning, the squat is the king of all weightlifting exercises and stands atop in its ability to maximize athletic potential. The squat stimulates optimal physical growth and development by strengthening the body's power base (quadriceps, gluteals, hamstrings, and abdominals). The biomechanics of the squat are similar to most power thrust movements from the hip and thigh area in baseball. This powerful thrust is required in running, jumping, throwing, and hitting.

Focus: The large muscle groups in the body's power zone—the lower back, hips, buttocks, and thighs

Procedure:

1. Position the bar across the shoulders with the load distributed over the mass of your back.

2. Position your hands comfortably about shoulder-width apart on the bar.

3. Keep your head up, chest out, shoulders back, and back flat with an arch at the base.

4. Keep your feet flat on the floor and spaced wider than shoulder-width with your toes turned out slightly.

5. Slowly bend your knees and descend under control until your upper legs are parallel to the floor with your back straight and your butt thrust back. Now rise back up in an explosive but controlled manner. If you're unable to squat completely parallel, go as far as possible, always maintaining proper posture.

Variations: You can also use dumbbells for resistance. Hold dumbbells at sides and squat.

Repetitions: 8 to 12 controlled, 3 to 4 sets

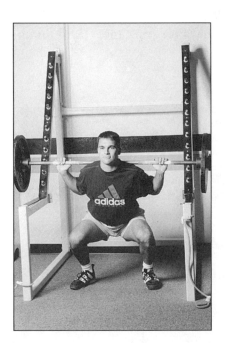 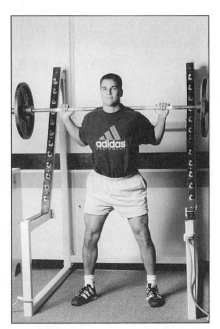

LUNGE

The lunge is an excellent core exercise to work single-leg strength and prevent strength imbalances. Several movements in baseball occur away from the center of the body. Pitching, throwing, and hitting all place the body with higher percentages of weight on a single leg at one point due to the weight shift involved in these skills. Obviously, running also involves single-leg control and strength.

Focus: Gluteals, hip flexors, quadriceps, hamstrings

Procedure:

1. Use the same placement of bar and alignment of the chest, shoulder, and back as in the squat.

2. Step forward with one leg.

3. Bend your knee and lower your body down.

4. Keep chest behind your knee and your knee behind your ankle.

5. Explosively push back to starting position and then work other leg.

Variations: You can also use dumbbells for resistance. Hold dumbbells at sides and lunge.

Repetitions: 8 to 12 controlled, 3 to 4 sets

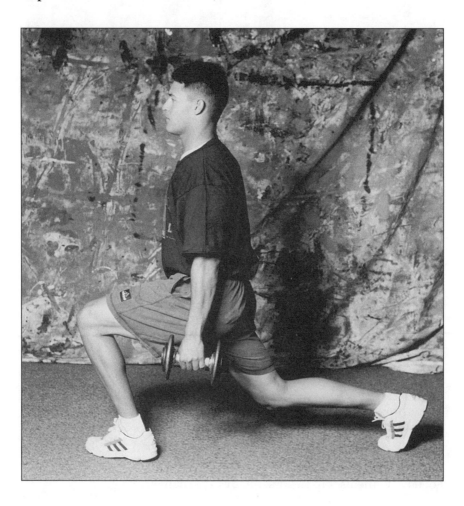

LEG PRESS

The leg press is a great exercise to alternate with the squat. It works the entire hip, thigh, and buttocks area with less emphasis on the lower back. The leg press is great for working the hip flexor region.

Focus: Quadriceps, hamstrings, gluteals

Procedure:

1. Lie or sit with your back flat against the pad and your feet secure against the platform.
2. Bend your knees and lower your weight slowly until your knees are at about a 90-degree angle.
3. Press up explosively back to the starting position.

Repetitions: 8 to 12 controlled, 3 to 4 sets

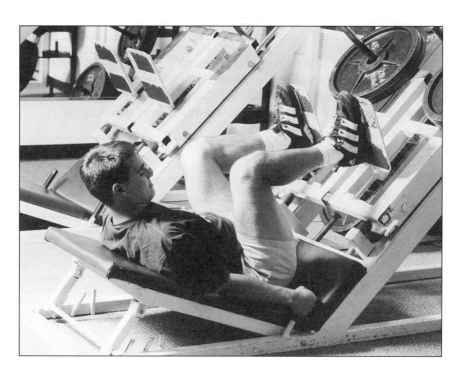

LEG EXTENSIONS

Leg extensions target the muscle group involved in any activity in which the leg is extended, including running and jumping movements common in baseball.

Focus: Quadriceps

Procedure:

1.   In a seated position, with your leg bent and feet secure against the pads, extend your knee until your lower leg is parallel to the floor.
2.   Slowly lower to the starting position.

Repetitions: 8 to 12 controlled, 3 to 4 sets

LEG CURL

Leg curls work the hamstrings, one of the most often injured muscles in sports. It's necessary to allow sufficient time to increase strength in this area. The hamstrings are crucial to the powerful contraction of leg extensions and vital to all jumping and quick start movements.

Focus: Hamstrings

Procedure:

1.   Lie face down with your legs extended and the backs of your heels against the pads.
2.   Grasp the handles to stabilize your body during the exercise.
3.   Lift your legs upward until the back of the pads are touching your buttocks.
4.   Return to the starting position.

Repetitions: 8 to 12 controlled, 3 to 4 sets

BACK REGION

The upper and lower back play key roles in baseball as they are involved in all throwing and swinging actions. The back makes up a huge muscle group that includes the rhomboids, latissimus dorsi, rotator cuff group, trapezius, and rear deltoid. Neglecting this group will leave you weak and open to injury. The muscles of the back provide the agonist/ antagonist balance for all major pressing and pulling actions.

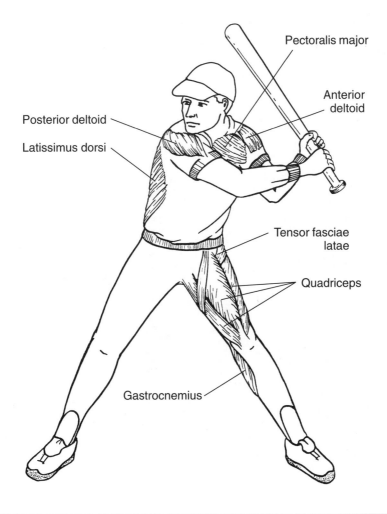

Back and leg muscles used in hitting.

LAT PULLDOWN

Focus: The upper portions of the latissimus dorsi (the muscles that fan out from your arm pits to midback)

Procedure:

1. Grasp the lat pulldown bar with hands slightly wider than shoulder-width apart.

2. Pull the bar straight down until it touches the front of your upper chest.

3. Return to original position and repeat.

Variations: Use the same mechanics but pull down to the base of your neck or lean back and pull to the bottom part of your chest.

Repetitions: 8 to 12 controlled, 3 to 4 sets

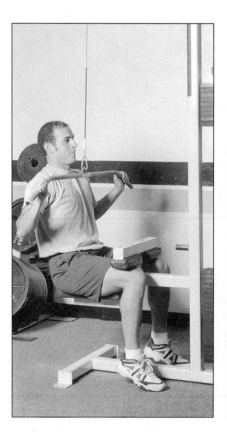 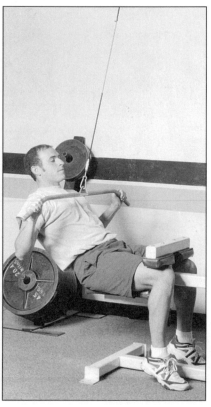

GOOD MORNING BENDS

This exercise targets the lower back muscles, which are vital to hitting, throwing, and balance.

Focus: Lower back region

Procedure:

1. Stand with your feet shoulder-width apart and the barbell behind your neck, resting on your shoulders.

2. Bend forward at the waist until your upper torso is parallel to the floor. As you bend forward, slightly bend your knees.

3. Return to starting position.

4. It's important to start with light weights. Do not jerk to assist movement. Keep your head up at all times.

Repetitions: 8 to 12 controlled, 3 to 4 sets

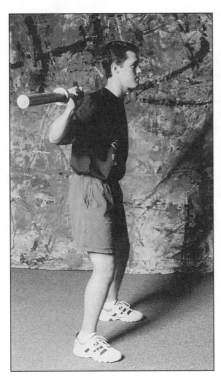
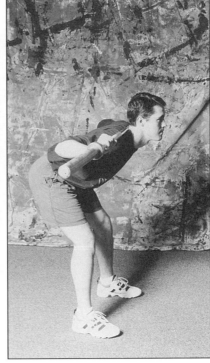

SEATED ROW

Focus: Lower back

Procedure:

1. Take a seated position with your knees slightly bent.
2. Grab the handle firmly and row to the chest area.
3. Straighten your back, pause, and return to the starting position.

Repetitions: 8 to 12 controlled, 3 to 4 sets

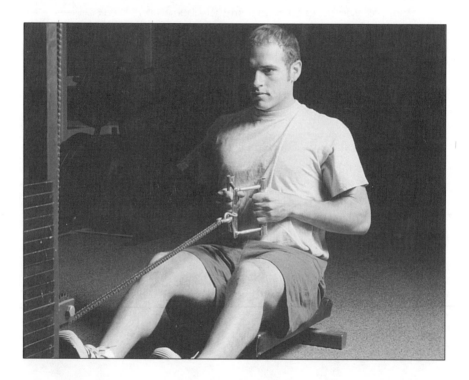

Abdominals

For a baseball player, strong abdominals are a must. Since baseball involves rotational movements in the trunk and abdominal region, this area must have exceptional strength. Strong abdominals also help prevent lower back injuries. Train the abdominals often and their recovery time will be minimal.

MEDICINE BALL TOSS

Focus: Upper abdominals, lower back

Procedure:

1. Bend your knees at a 90-degree angle and have a partner lightly stand on your toes.

2. From a lying position, holding the medicine ball, sit up with abdominals contracted and toss the ball to your partner.

3. Catch the ball from your partner in an upright position.

4. With abdominals contracted, return to the starting position and repeat the exercise.

Repetitions: 20 to 25 with a nine-pound medicine ball

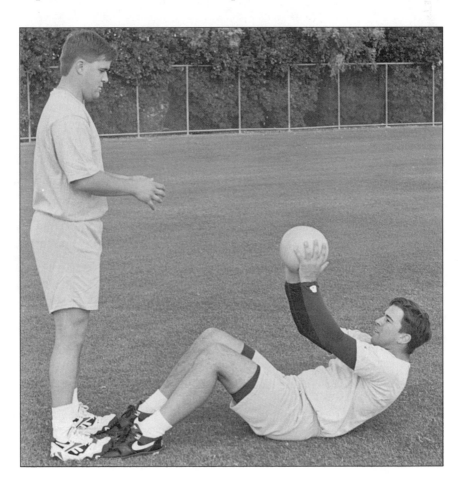

JACKKNIFE SIT-UP

Focus: Abdominal wall and lower back

Procedure:

1. Lying on your back, bring your legs straight up to an L position.
2. With the medicine ball on your chest, press up to your toes, bringing your shoulders off the ground.
3. Hold at the top for one second, then return to starting position and repeat.

Repetitions: 20 to 25 with a nine-pound medicine ball

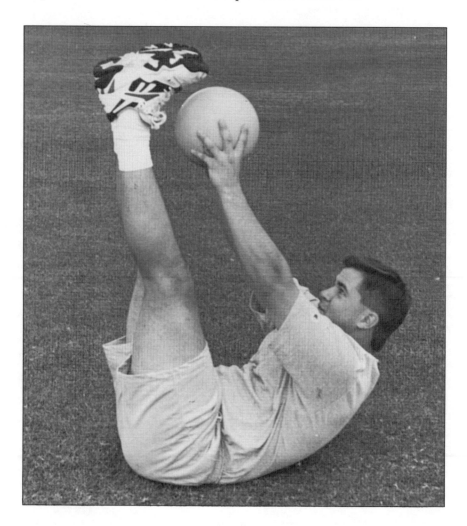

RUSSIAN TWISTS

Focus: Oblique musculature (side abdominal muscles)

Proceedure:

1. With knees bent, grasp a medicine ball firmly and extend it out in front of your chest.

2. Bring your back off the ground about halfway toward your knees.

3. Hold this position and in a quick, controlled fashion rotate the abdominals and trunk area.

Repetitions: 20 to 25 with a nine-pound medicine ball

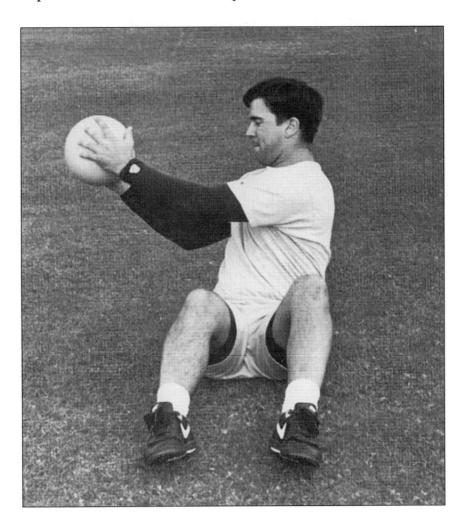

HEEL TOUCHES

Focus: Oblique musculature

Procedure:

1.   Lie with your shoulders flat, knees bent, and heels together.

2.   With both hands starting on the chest area, bring your shoulder blades off the ground about six inches and hold this position.

3.   With your right hand, reach around and touch your right heel and return to your chest.

4.   Proceed with your left hand to left heel.

Repetitions: 20 to 25

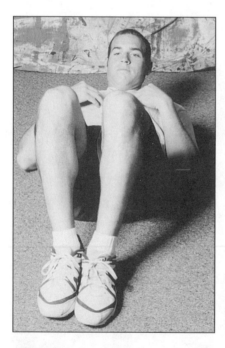 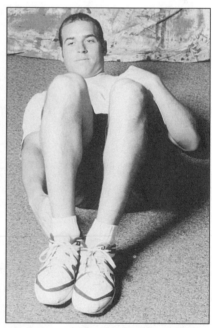

CHEST

The pectoral area plays an instrumental role in throwing and hitting and is needed for keeping good balance with the back for good upper body strength. Core presses that work the chest coupled with core upper back exercises also greatly improve shoulder joint stability.

BENCH PRESS

Focus: Chest area

Procedure:

1. Lie flat on a bench with your feet securely on the ground at either side.
2. Grasp the bar with an overhand grip just a little wider than shoulder-width.
3. Lower the bar with control to your chest, then press upward.
4. Variations include the incline bench press for the upper chest area and the decline bench press for the lower chest.

Repetitions: 8 to 12, 3 to 4 sets

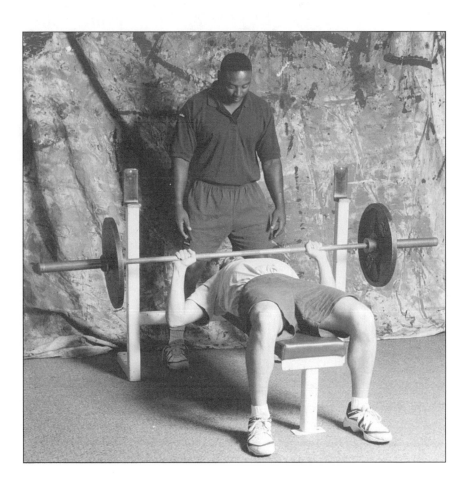

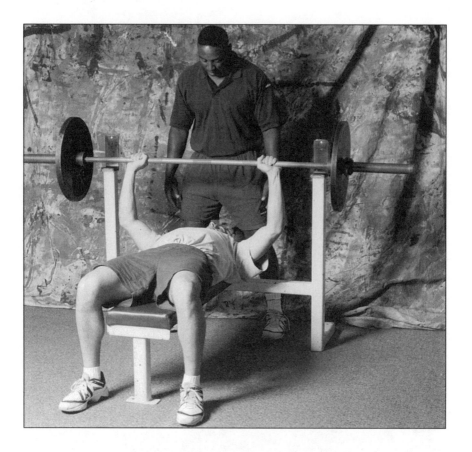

DUMBBELL BENCH PRESS

This is a great variation of the traditional bench press. Dumbbells really emphasize muscle balance.

Focus: Overall chest area

Procedure:

1. Lie flat on a bench with your feet secure on ground on either side.
2. Grasp the dumbbells with an overhand grip.
3. Balance each dumbbell and lower until parallel with your chest, then press upward.

Variations: Try performing these with incline and decline bench positions.

Repetitions: 8 to 12, 3 to 4 sets

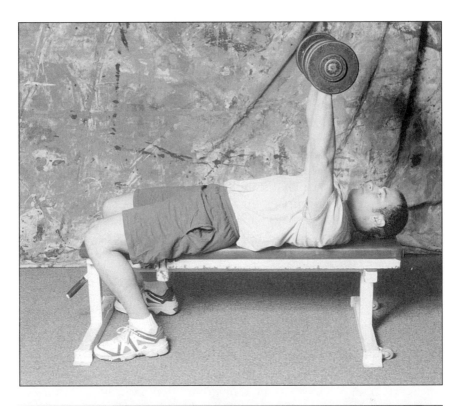

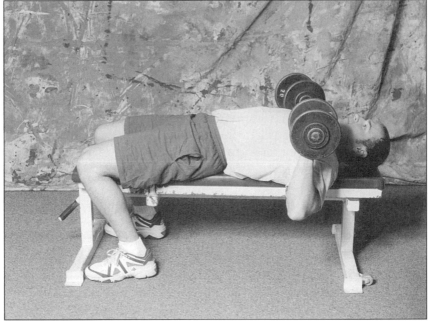

SHOULDER

The shoulders make up a very large and powerful muscle group that assists in almost all upper body movements. The deltoid and rhomboid muscles that make up the bulk of the shoulder area are powerful, dense muscles seldom injured in baseball. It's the smaller muscle groups in the rotator cuff area that are more susceptible to injury.

The shoulder joint area is one of the most complex regions of the body because it's able to perform multiple movements, which is quite amazing for a joint with minimal stability. Sports like baseball that involve repetitive motions from this area increase chances of injury to the shoulder region. You should have a sound understanding of this area before working here to increase strength. Movements of the shoulder girdle include

adduction/abduction—horizontally, laterally, vertically;

internal/external rotation; and

flexion/extension.

The shoulder will perform many other movements, but these are the main areas we're concerned with. The muscles of the shoulder girdle conform around the scapula, a bone much like a small shallow saucer. The scapula allows for extreme range of motion. However, because of this freedom, the ligaments that keep the shoulder in place are relatively weak compared to the ligaments that help keep the hip in place. Stability comes from muscles and tendons running across the joint and a small rim of cartilage that increases the depth of the socket. These must be maintained with flexibility and strength work to help prevent injury. Large muscles in the shoulder area and the arm, deltoid rhomboid, triceps, biceps, and latissimus dorsi help to stabilize the shoulder.

Four small but very important muscles that make up the rotator cuff along with their tendons are the subscapular, supraspinous, infraspinous, and teres minor. This group is located on the rear of the scapula or shoulder blade. Neglecting these small muscle groups in a strength-training program would be detrimental to a baseball player. Common imbalances of front deltoid muscles and the weakness of these small muscles is one of the major reasons for chronic and acute arm problems.

These muscles cannot be isolated through conventional shoulder exercises. To maximize conditioning of this area, you need to use specific exercises with light weights and tubing. We strongly recommend that baseball players warm up this area before starting their weight program. Do the tubing exercises for the shoulder three to four times a week as part of your warm-up before weight training. As we approach the core exercises for the shoulder, you'll see that we avoid heavy weight pressing specifically for the shoulder. As mentioned before, the shoulder area is involved in almost all upper body movements, so it gets its fair share of the work. We want to avoid the big imbalance often achieved between the front deltoid and the posterior deltoid.

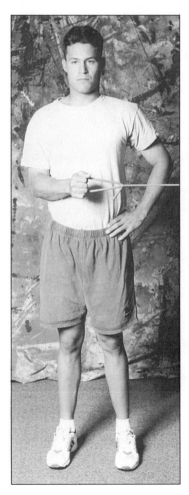 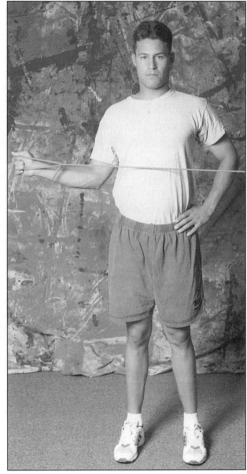

Shoulder Joint Warm-Up Tubing Exercises

External rotation at 0-degree abduction: Standing with the involved elbow flexed 90 degrees at your side and the involved arm across the front of your body, grip the tubing handle with the other end of the tubing fixed straight ahead, and pull with your arm, keeping your elbow at your side. Return tubing slowly, with control.

Internal rotation at 0-degree abduction: Stand with your elbow at your side flexed 90 degrees and your shoulder rotated out. Grip the tubing handle with the other end of the tubing fixed straight ahead, and pull your arm across your body, keeping your elbow at your side. Return tubing slowly, with control.

External rotation at 90-degree abduction (slow): Stand with your shoulder abducted 90 degrees and your elbow flexed 90 degrees. Grip the tubing handle with the other end of the tubing fixed straight behind and, keeping your shoulder abducted, rotate your shoulder back, keeping your elbow at 90 degrees. Return tubing and hand to start position slowly, with control.

Internal rotation at 90-degree abduction (slow): Stand with your shoulder abducted to 90 degrees, externally rotated 90 degrees, and elbow flexed 90 degrees. Grip the tubing handle with the other end of the tubing fixed straight behind. Keeping your shoulder abducted, rotate the shoulder forward, keeping your elbow at 90 degrees. Return tubing and hand to start position slowly, with control.

Diagonal pattern (D1) flexion: Gripping tubing handle in the hand of the involved arm, begin with your arm out from your side 45 degrees and your palm facing backward. After turning your palm forward, flex your elbow and bring your arm up and over the uninvolved shoulder. Turn your palm down and reverse to take your arm to starting position. Perform this exercise with control.

Diagonal pattern (D2) flexion: With the involved hand, grip the tubing handle across your body and against the thigh of your opposite-side leg. Starting with your palm down, rotate the palm up to begin. Proceed to flex elbow and bring your arm up and over the involved shoulder, with your palm facing inward. Turn the palm down and reverse to take your arm to starting position. Perform this exercise with control.

Diagonal pattern (D2) extension: The involved hand grips the tubing handle overhead and out to the side. Pull the tubing down and across your body to the opposite side of your leg. During the motion, lead with your thumb.

Repetitions: 15 to 20 for each arm for each exercise

SHRUGS

Focus: Entire shoulder area

Procedure:

1. Hold a barbell or dumbbells with an overhand grip extended down in front of your body.

2. Lift your shoulders up in a circular motion.

3. Lower and repeat motion.

Repetitions: 10 to 15, 3 to 4 sets

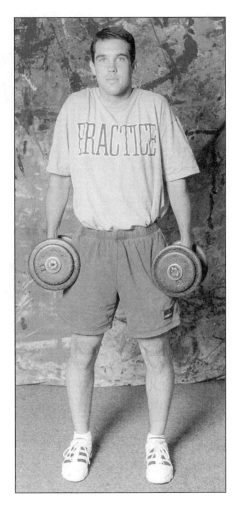

LATERAL RAISE

Focus: Medial head of deltoid

Procedure:

1. Grasp a dumbbell extended down by your side with an overhand grip.
2. Raise the dumbbells laterally to shoulder height with your arms parallel to the ground and your palms facing down. Keep your elbows soft or slightly bent to reduce elbow stress.
3. Lower back to your side and repeat.

Repetitions: 10 to 15, 3 to 4 sets

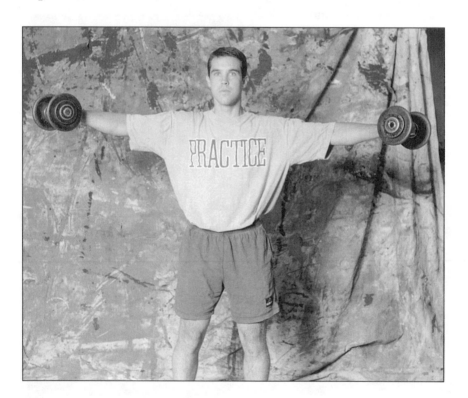

DUMBELL MILITARY PRESS

Focus: Entire shoulder area

Procedure:

1. Seated on a bench with back support, start with the barbell at the top of your chest area.

2. Press the bar above your head, not quite locking your arms.

3. Lower the weight and repeat.

Variations: You can also do this exercise with a dumbbell. To perform a behind-the-neck press, lower the weight behind your head to the base of your neck and extend up.

Repetitions: 10 to 15, 3 to 4 sets

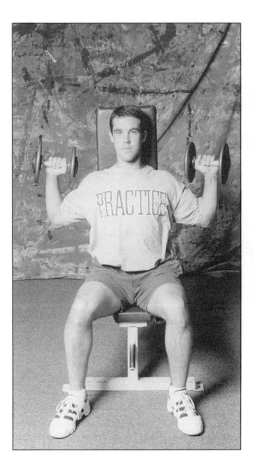
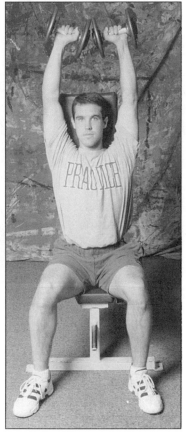

AUXILIARY MUSCLES

So far we've focused on the core area of the muscles—the legs, back, abdominals, chest, and shoulders. Now we'll turn our attention to the smaller, secondary muscles of the upper body: the biceps, triceps, and forearms. Building these muscles appeals to many young lifters who want to acquire the "big guns" of a Juan Gonzales or Jose Canseco. Yet, young players need to be reminded that such arms are built over years of intense conditioning and training and that as impressive as arm size can be, what's more important is to achieve optimal proportions and strength throughout the core region—this is where Gonzales's and Canseco's power really comes from. The smaller muscle groups alone provide a minimal amount of power. Rather, these smaller muscle groups assist the larger muscles when lifting and playing baseball.

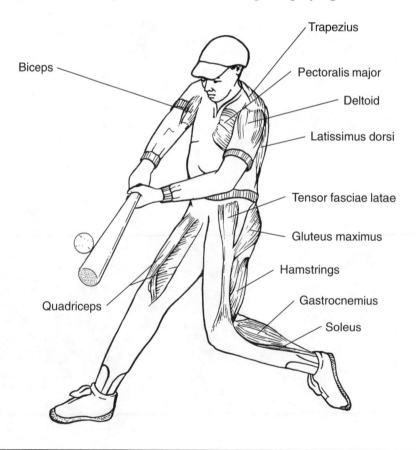

Muscles used in midswing.

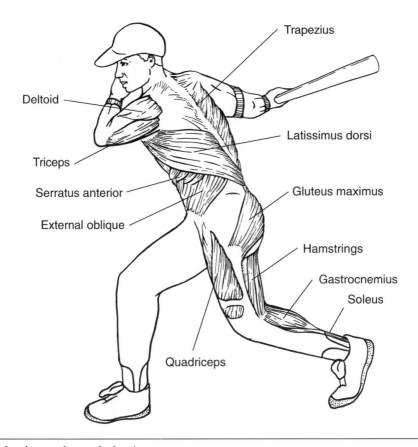

Deltoid

Triceps

Serratus anterior

External oblique

Quadriceps

Trapezius

Latissimus dorsi

Gluteus maximus

Hamstrings

Gastrocnemius

Soleus

Muscles used at end of swing.

When the core area is worked in a strength-training program, the small muscles also receive quality amounts of work. For this reason, when planning a workout, the multijoint or core exercises should be performed first, followed by the single joint (secondary) exercises. Because if you perform triceps extensions before the bench press, for example, you will not be able to handle as much weight on the bench press. The secondary exercises, such as triceps extensions, are usually single-joint movements that isolate a particular muscle group. They are very taxing to a particular muscle and will decrease that muscle's work output when you need it to assist the larger muscles. We recommend a combination of multijoint and single-joint exercises. Below are some auxiliary exercises for good body balance. Incorporating these exercises into your workouts will be discussed in the Combination Training Drills chapter (chapter 10).

CALF RAISES

Calf raises along with the leg extension and leg curl exercises presented earlier help strengthen the auxiliary muscles of the leg and hip region.

Focus: Calves

Procedure:

1. Place the front half of your feet on a raised platform with your feet shoulder-width apart.

2. Raise up on your toes, squeezing your calf muscles at top.

3. Return to starting position. This exercise can be varied to hit different parts of the calf by pointing toes out or in.

Repetitions: 20 to 30, 3 to 4 sets

PREACHER CURLS

Focus: Biceps

Procedure:

1. Seated at the preacher bench with a bar held in an underhand grip, extend your arms straight down—do not lock your elbows.

2. Slowly raise the bar to your shoulders.

3. Return to starting position

Repetitions: 8 to 12, 3 to 4 sets

STANDING STRAIGHT BAR CURLS

Focus: Biceps

Procedure:

1. Stand with your feet shoulder-width apart grasping the bar with an underhand grip.

2. Begin with your arms extended below your waist and slowly lift the weight up to your shoulders by bending your elbows.

3. Slowly return to starting position, being careful not to lock your elbows.

Repetitions: 8 to 12, 3 to 4 sets

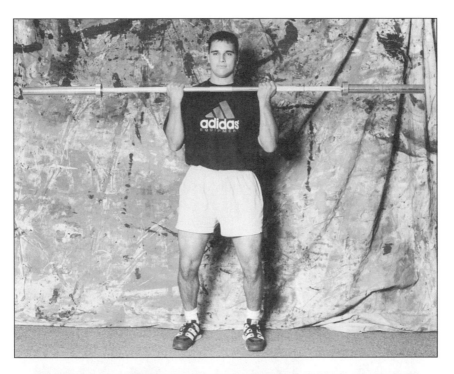

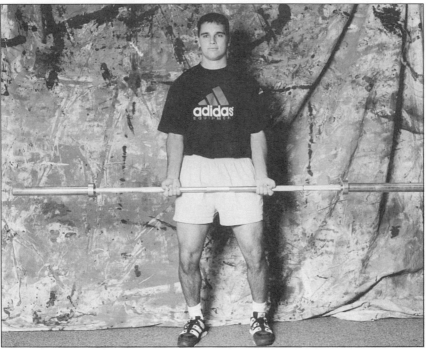

ALTERNATING DUMBBELL CURLS

Focus: Biceps

Procedure:

1. Sit or stand with your feet together and knees slightly bent, with a dumbbell in each hand in an underhand grip at your sides.

2. Slowly raise one dumbbell in front of your body to your shoulder, keeping your elbow tight to your body.

3. Slowly return to starting position and repeat with your other arm.

Repetitions: 8 to 12 each side, 3 to 4 sets

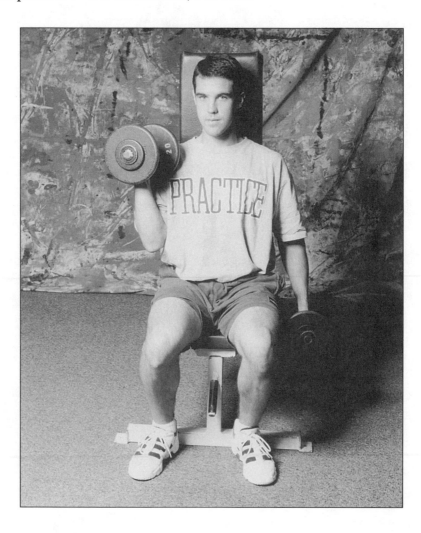

LYING TRICEPS EXTENSIONS

Focus: Triceps

Procedure:

1. Lying on a bench, grasp a bar in an overhand grip slightly less than shoulder-width apart and raise the weight directly above your chest so your arms are straight. Do not lock your elbows.

2. Keeping your elbows stationary, bend your arms and lower your hands to your forehead.

3. Return to starting position.

Repetitions: 8 to 12, 3 to 4 sets

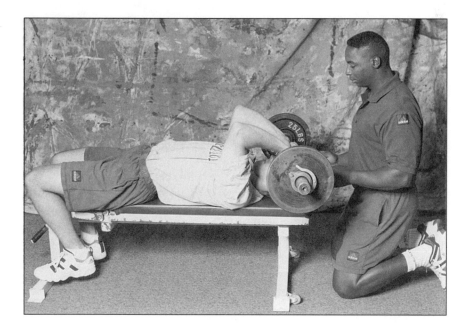

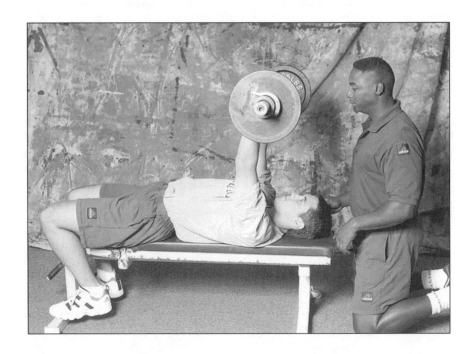

TRICEPS PUSHDOWN

Focus: Triceps

Procedure:

1. Standing with your feet shoulder-width apart, grasp a bar in an overhand grip. Keeping your elbows tight to your body, push the bar straight down so your arms are extended—do not lock your elbows.

2. Keeping your elbows stationary, bend your arms until the bar reaches your lower chest.

3. Return to starting position

Repetitions: 8 to 12, 3 to 4 sets

TRICEPS KICKBACKS

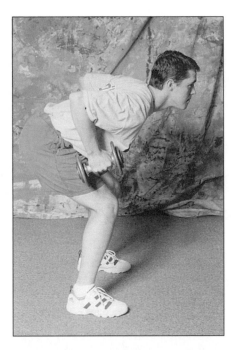

Focus: Triceps

Procedure:

1. Standing with your feet shoulder-width apart, knees slightly bent and leaning forward, hold a dumbbell in each hand in an overhand grip.

2. With your back straight and the dumbbell held at a 90-degree angle at the side of your body with your elbow up, extend your arm straight back, keeping your elbow stationary.

3. Return to starting position.

Repetitions: 8 to 12 on each side, 3 to 4 sets

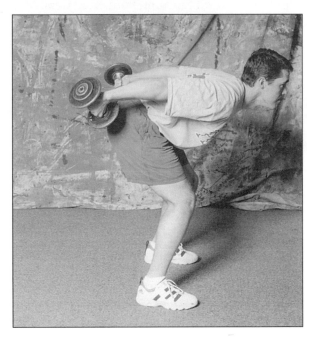

WRIST ROLLS

Focus: Forearms

Procedure:

1. Stand with a free weight attached to a bar held in an overhand grip in front of your body with your arms straight.

2. Slowly lower the bar moving your wrists only.

3. Return to starting position.

Repetitions: 15 to 20, 3 to 4 sets

HAMMER STRENGTH WORK

Focus: Forearms and biceps

Procedure:

1. Sit at a preacher bench with a dumbbell in each hand in an overhand grip with your knuckles facing in. Extend your arms straight down.

2. Slowly raise both dumbbells until touching your shoulders.

3. Return to starting position.

Repetitions: 8 to 12, 3 to 4 sets

BARBELL WRIST CURLS

Focus: Forearms

Procedure:

1. Sit with arms resting on knees and a barbell held in an underhand grip.

2. Slowly lower the bar moving your wrists only.

3. Return to starting position.

Repetitions: 15 to 20, 3 to 4 sets

CHAPTER 5

APPLICATION OF STRENGTH TRAINING

If you look back on the history of

weight-training programs, you'll find that most methods were designed by power lifters, Olympic lifters, and body builders. But we understand as baseball players that we will not be effective if we train the same way a body builder or power lifter does—the demands of our sport are far different. Nonetheless, it will help us to know the various training methods and systems these athletes use. Lifters' proven track records of manipulating training variables and the muscle to bring optimal gains in size and strength are second to none.

We return to a question many have asked us: "What is a good strength-training program for my team or athlete?" There's no one answer to this question. Coaches and trainers need to understand various methods to help them choose the best program for their baseball players. Maximum gains in strength and size involve mixing various training programs and manipulating the weights and exercises accordingly.

The biggest problem with most conditioning programs is that they fall into a rut of one training system. Coaches forget about the specific needs analysis of certain athletes and apply a single system to the whole team for the duration of the season. This is a major mistake, as it inevitably leads to below-maximum gain for everyone and does not address the individuals' particular needs. Working within one system, players tend to lose focus quickly, and their muscles adapt to the training, leading to plateaus in strength gains. As discussed in chapter 4, for continuous improvement, workouts must impose a demand and a consistent change on the body system. Let's look at the different training methods and systems used most commonly to build strength and power.

CIRCUIT TRAINING

Circuit training along with multipurpose work stations became a popular and convenient form of training in the mid 1970s. Circuit training involves a series of weightlifting exercises performed one after the other with minimal rest (15 to 30 seconds) between exercises. The goal of the circuit program is to improve your cardiovascular condition and muscle mass. The limited rest between exercises allows the heart rate to remain elevated for the duration of the routine. This program's added appeal is that it's very efficient with large numbers of athletes or under time constraints.

With the rapid succession of exercises, the resistance is fairly low, at 40 to 70 percent of one's maximum. As you'll recall, this percent 1RM range builds muscle size rather than targeting improved strength. If circuit training is your only feasible means of weight training, then by all means do it. However, we do not recommend this method of training as your principal system. Except for the beginning of the strength phase (first two weeks), circuit training will not give you the strength gains you're looking for. The main reason for incorporating a circuit-training routine in baseball conditioning is to add variety to your workouts.

Circuit training is most effective during the in-season phase of your training cycle. It's a great method to incorporate into heavy core programs when working auxiliary muscles, as discussed in chapter 4. Circuit training can also be incorporated all through your conditioning program in segments to change or work small muscle groups. Large muscle groups cannot be worked in the circuit method, as they need proper rest to recuperate in order to work at the high levels needed for maximal strength gains. Again we come back to the percent 1RM necessary for optimal strength gains. Circuit training does not work above 70 percent 1RM, where strength increases noticeably occur. Greater size alone is not going to enhance your game as a baseball player. Table 5.1 provides a sample circuit schedule.

Table 5.1   Sample Circuit Schedule: Weeks 1-2

**Primary training focus: Muscle adaptation to training
and muscle endurance**

Muscle group	Exercise	Sets/reps	% max.	No. of days	Intensity
Chest	(choose from exercise option chart)	2-3/10-12	70	3	Low
Legs		2-3/10-12	70	3	Low
Back		2-3/10-12	70	3	Low
Back		2-3/10-12	70	3	Low
Shoulders		2-3/10-12	70	3	Low

Auxiliary circuit

Biceps		2-3/10-12	70	3	Low
Abdominals		2-3/20-25	—	3	Low
Triceps		2-3/10-12	70	3	Low

MULTIPLE-SET SYSTEM

Most training programs use a variation of the multiple-set principle. This method calls for two to three warm-up sets of increasing weight, followed by three to four sets of the same prescribed weight. Five to six reps per set offer optimal gains using this system. This is a very good method to employ when working the core area.

Multiple-set training is best implemented by focusing on two to three target areas per circuit training workout. For example, on Monday you might do chest and leg work, on Wednesday shoulder and back exercises, and on Friday triceps, abdominals, and back work (see table 5.2).

Table 5.2   Sample Multiple-Set Training Table

Day/muscle group	Exercise	No. of sets warm-up	% warm-up	No. of sets fixed work	% fixed work
Monday					
Chest		3-4		3-4	
			50-60		80-85
Leg		3-4		3-4	
Monday					
Chest					
Leg					
Wednesday					
Shoulders		3-4		3-4	
			50-60		80-85
Biceps		3-4		3-4	
Wednesday					
Shoulders					
Biceps					
Friday					
Back		3-4		3-4	
			50-60		80-85
Triceps		3-4		3-4	
Friday					
Back					
Triceps					

Note: This can be incorporated into the power or specific power-training phases for a portion of the prescribed number of weeks.

Super Setting

You're likely familiar with the super set method—also called the "beach biceps" workout—in which you rush into the weight room and start doing consecutive sets of various curl exercises to get the instant pump on your biceps. You conclude your workout by rolling up your sleeves and walking out of the gym, hoping someone will notice. The idea behind super setting is to work a muscle group more intensely by challenging it with at least two different exercises performed in succession. The initial exercise exhausts the muscle, then the second one places a new demand on it, making it work harder. While this is one of the best

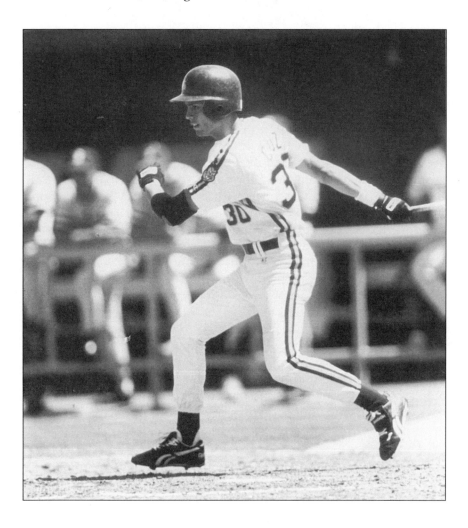

methods for increasing muscle size (but not maximum strength), the merit of super setting for baseball players is to help break up tedious workout ruts and really shock the muscle. A different type of stimulation to the muscles from time to time is healthy for muscle and strength growth. After the initial strength phase of your program is completed, we recommend doing super sets every three to four weeks in your training cycle. This adds variety and a new challenge for your muscles. Use super sets for one whole body revolution.

Example: Monday—Legs and back
             Wednesday—Chest and biceps
             Friday—Triceps and shoulders

Push-Pull Method

A great method to train opposing muscle groups, both large and small, is the push-pull method. Opposing muscle groups include upper back and chest, triceps and biceps, and the lower back and abdominals. Try using this method along with multiple-set training to maximize the work to large muscles on heavy training days. You can divide the core area into various body parts and hit both parts hard without the fatigue factor affecting or diminishing the work for the other part. This technique has an injury prevention benefit, as well. When you work opposing muscle groups together, you stretch one muscle group while the other works. Studies have shown this method can help prevent excessive stress and strain of the muscle.

The harmony of the muscle groups working together is also great for maximal strength gains. The push-pull is a very efficient method for large muscle groups and provides opportunity for high amounts of work for the core area in less time. An example of the push-pull method is working the chest and back together. Working the chest pushes your arms away from your body. The back is then worked with a pull that brings your arms toward your body. You should use this method with all opposing muscle groups using a variety of combinations. For example, pull with your biceps and push with your triceps; pull with your back and push with your shoulders; and so on.

Pyramid Program

The pyramid program, which has several variations, is one of the most widely used training methods today and is believed to be the best system for increasing strength. We practice the pyramid system for the majority of our strength training program (60 to 70 percent). Two basic objectives of the pyramid system are increasing the intensity of each lift while decreasing the number of repetitions.

The pyramid is set up to overload the muscles as much as possible with the fewest number of reps. Your pyramid can be set up to meet any number of repetitions as long as the weight is being increased. In our program, we usually cap our pyramid with 3-rep maximums. A pyramid starts with a set of light weight of 10 to 12 repetitions. With each set, the weight is increased and repetitions are decreased until you reach your prescribed maximum. Then you work your way back down the pyramid, decreasing the weight. Finish with a set of 10 to 12 repetitions. A full pyramid consists of both the upward climb of the pyramid and the descent of the pyramid.

PERIODIZATION

In chapter 1 we explained the periodization phases for baseball, which include regeneration, strength, power, specific power, preseason, and in-season. Table 5.3 is a sample periodization chart. Use this program chart to periodize your training seasons. Remember, you can use this as a guideline for the number of weeks available to you or your team. For percentages, see table 4.1, the Maximum Lift Chart, on pages 42-46 in chapter 4.

Table 5.3   Periodization Table

Phase	No. of days/ week	No. of sets	No. of reps	%max.	Intensity	No. of weeks
Regeneration	3-5	NA	NA	NA	Low	3-8
Strength	3	3	10-12	70	Low	2
Power	3	3-4	6-8	80-85	High	4
Specific power	3	4	1-4	85-90	Very high	2-3
Preseason	2-3	2	12-15	65-70	Low	1-2
In-season	2-3	2	12-15	65-70	Low	Season

Use table 5.4 as a guide to identify specific muscle groups and areas. Use table 5.5 to identify specific exercises with muscle groups.

Table 5.4 Specific Areas and Muscle Groups

Focus area	Primary muscle groups	
Legs—front	Quadriceps group: •Vastus lateralis •Vastus intermedius Adductor group Abductor group	•Vastus medialis •Rectus femoris
Legs—back	Hamstrings group: •Biceps femoris Gluteus group	•Semitendinosous
Back	Latissimus dorsi Middle and lower trapezius Rhomboid Spinal erector	
Chest	Pectoralis major Anterior deltoid Pectoralis minor	
Shoulders	Upper trapezius Anterior deltoid Pectoralis minor	

Focus area	Secondary muscle groups
Arms	Biceps Triceps Forearm
Calves	Gastrocnemius Soleus

Table 5.5 Exercise Option Chart

Focus	Core/major lift	Secondary/complementary lift
Legs	Leg press Squats Lunges	Leg curls Leg extensions Calf raises

(continued)

Focus	Core/major lift	Secondary/complementary lift
	Hack squat	Adductor machine
	Step-ups	Abductor machine
Back	Seated row	One-arm rows
	Lat pulldown	Pull-ups
	Bent-over row	Back extensions
	Good morning bends	
Chest	Bench press	Dumbbell bench press– flat/incline
	Incline bench press	Dumbbell fly– flat/incline
	Decline bench press	Pec dec
		Push-ups
Shoulder	Shoulder press	Front deltoid raise
	Shrugs	Side deltoid raise
	Plate raises	Rear deltoid raise
Arms	Biceps curl–barbell	Triceps pushdowns
	Dumbbells curl– incline/seated	Triceps kickbacks
	Preacher curl	Triceps extensions
	Concentration curl	Seated dips
	Hammer curl	Wrist rolls
Abdominals	Medicine ball toss	
	Jackknife sit-ups	
	Russian twists	
	Heel touches	

Weight-Training Guidelines to Prevent Injury

1. **Avoid incorrect technique.** The most common injuries during weightlifting are caused by incorrect technique. When lifting weights, work to become as proficient and precise as possible when performing the exercises.

2. **Use the right amount of weight.** The higher you go up in weight, the higher the risk potential of injury. Proper control of the

(continued)

weight as you lower it and push it up must be maintained within its biomechanical boundaries at all times.

3.   **Avoid overtraining.** Overtraining affects the body's overall level of strength and conditioning. Proper rest to restore the body's energy sources will help in the recovery and growth phases of training.

4.   **Warm up and stretch properly.** Proper warm-up and stretching help to relax and elongate the muscle and make it alert neurologically and more pliable and less susceptible to injury.

5.   **Eat nutritiously.** Heavy training accompanied by improper dieting can also lead to injury. Remember proper nutrition is the fuel for growth, strength, and energy.

6.   **Concentrate.** You need to stay focused. Allowing yourself to be distracted or preoccupied during a workout is an invitation to injury. Focus on your training and train smart.

Strength Phase

The strength phase is designed to reacquaint your body to strength training (see table 5.6, a-b). This phase is crucial, as it is the foundation of your overall strength-building program. Note that during the first two weeks a total body format is used. These two weeks help serve as a muscle conditioner stage and prepare the body with six lifts before the power phase, when the body will be broken into smaller body segments for the subsequent workouts.

Table 5.6a   Sample Strength Phase Chart: Week 1

Day/ week 1	Exercise	Station no.	No. of sets	Reps	% max.
Monday	Bench press	1	3	15, 12, 10	See table 5.3.
	Squats	2	3	15, 12, 10	
	Biceps curls	3	3	15, 12, 10	
	Lateral raise	4	3	15, 12, 10	
	Lat pulldown	5	3	15, 12, 10	

(continued)

Table 5.6a   Sample Strength Phase Chart: Week 1   *(continued)*

Day/ week 1	Exercise	Station no.	No. of sets	Reps	% max.
	Triceps press	6	3	15, 12, 10	
Wednesday	Incline bench press	1	3	15, 12, 10	
	Leg press	2	3	15, 12, 10	
	Straight bar curls	3	3	15, 12, 10	
	Shoulder press	4	3	15, 12, 10	
	Pull-ups	5	3	15, 12, 10	
	Triceps pushdowns	6	3	15, 12, 10	
Friday	Dumbbell bench press	1	3	15, 12, 10	
	Lunges	2	3	15, 12, 10	
	Preacher curls	3	3	15, 12, 10	
	Shrugs	4	3	15, 12, 10	
	Seated rows	5	3	15, 12, 10	
	Triceps kickbacks	6	3	15, 12, 10	

Table 5.6b   Sample Strength Phase Chart: Week 2

Day/ week 2	Exercise	Station no.	No. of sets	Reps	% max.
Monday	Step-ups/ leg extension	1	3	15, 12, 10	See table 5.3.
	Incline curls/ wrist rolls	2	3	15, 12, 10	
	Lat pulldown/ seated rows	3	3	15, 12, 10	
	Bench press/ pec dec	4	3	15, 12, 10	

(continued)

Table 5.6b   Sample Strength Phase Chart: Week 2   (*continued*)

Day/ week 2	Exercise	Station no.	No. of sets	Reps	% max.
Monday	Shrugs/rear deltoid	5	3	15, 12, 10	See table 5.3.
	Pushdowns/ kickbacks	6	3	15, 12, 10	
Wednesday	Squats/leg curls	1	3	15, 12, 10	
	Russian twist/ heel touches	2	3	25, 25, 25	
	Forearms	3	3	25, 25, 25	
	One-arm rows	4	3	15, 12, 10	
	Triceps extension	5	3	15, 12, 10	
Friday	Dumbbell bench press	1	3	15, 12, 10	
	Lunges/leg extension	2	3	15, 12, 10	
	Preacher curls	3	3	15, 12, 10	
	Shrugs	4	3	15, 12, 10	
	Seated rows	5	3	15, 12, 10	
	Abdominals	6	3	15, 12, 10	

Power Phase

The power phase focuses on increasing strength and power. Specific muscle groups used in baseball such as the gluteals, shoulders, and arm muscles are targeted during this phase. Specific body parts are worked on certain days (add weight accordingly). Follow the program chart (table 5.7, a-e) for the specific power phase and preseason phase. For weeks 4 through 7, see table 5.5, the Exercise Option Chart, for choice of exercises. Additional abdominal exercises are presented in chapter 9.

Table 5.7a   Sample Power Phase Chart: Week 3

Day/week 3	Exercise	Station no.	No. of sets	Reps	% max.
Monday	Bench press	1	3	10, 8, 6	See table 5.3.
	Pec dec	2	3	10, 10, 8	
	Squats	3	3	10, 8, 6	
	Leg curls	4	3	10, 10, 8	
	Bar dips	5	3	10, 10, 10	
	Abdominal work	6	3	10, 10, 8	
	Forearm work	7	3	25, 25, 25	
	Leg press	8	3	25, 25, 25	
Wednesday	Seated rows	1	3	10, 8, 6	
	One-arm rows	2	3	10, 10, 8	
	Preacher curls	3	3	10, 10, 8	
	Seated dumbbell curls	4	3	10, 10, 8	
	Lat pulldown	5	3	10, 10, 8	
	Hammer curls	6	3	10, 10, 8	
	Abdominal work	7	3	25, 25, 25	
Friday	Dumbbell military press	1	3	10, 8, 6	
	Side lateral raise	2	3	10, 10, 8	
	Triceps extension	3	3	10, 8, 6	
	Triceps kickbacks	4	3	10, 8, 6	
	Shrugs	5	3	15, 12, 10	
	Triceps pushdowns	6	3	10, 10, 8	
	Abdominal work	7	3	25, 25, 25	
	Forearm work	8	3	25, 25, 25	

Table 5.7b   Sample Power Phase Chart: Week 4

Day/ week 4	Exercise	Station no.	No. of sets	Reps	% max.
Monday	Legs: core lift	1	3	10, 8, 6	See table 5.3
	Legs: auxiliary	2	3	10, 10, 8	
	Shoulders: core	3	3	10, 8, 6	
	Shoulders: auxiliary	4	3	10, 10, 8	
	Legs: core lift	5	3	10, 10, 10	
	Shoulders: auxiliary	6	3	10, 10, 8	
	Forearm work	7	3	25, 25, 25	
	Abdominal work	8	3	25, 25, 25	
Wednesday	Chest: core lift	1	3	10, 8, 6	
	Chest: auxiliary	2	3	10, 10, 8	
	Biceps: core	3	3	10, 10, 8	
	Biceps: auxiliary	4	3	10, 10, 8	
	Abdominal work	5	3	25, 25, 25	
Friday	Back: core	1	3	10, 8, 6	
	Back: auxiliary	2	3	10, 10, 8	
	Triceps	3	3	10, 8, 6	
	Triceps	4	3	10, 8, 6	
	Back: core	5	3	15, 12, 10	
	Triceps	6	3	10, 10, 8	
	Abdominal work	7	3	25, 25, 25	
	Forearm work	8	3	25, 25, 25	

Table 5.7c   Sample Power Phase Chart: Week 5

Day/ week 5	Exercise	Station no.	No. of sets	Reps	% max.
Monday	Legs: core lift	1	3	8, 8, 6	See table 5.3.
	Legs: auxiliary	2	3	10, 10, 8	
	Shoulders: core	3	3	8, 8, 6	
	Shoulders: auxiliary	4	3	10, 10, 8	
	Legs: core lift	5	3	10, 6, 6	
	Shoulders: auxiliary	6	3	10, 10, 8	
	Forearm work	7	3	25, 25, 25	
	Abdominal work	8	3	25, 25, 25	
Wednesday	Chest: core lift	1	3	8, 8, 6	
	Chest: auxiliary	2	3	10, 10, 8	
	Biceps: core	3	3	10, 6, 6	
	Biceps: auxiliary	4	3	10, 10, 8	
	Abdominal work	5	3	25, 25, 25	
Friday	Back: core	1	3	8, 8, 6	
	Back: auxiliary	2	3	10, 10, 8	
	Triceps	3	3	10, 6, 6	
	Triceps	4	3	10, 8, 6	
	Back: core	5	3	8, 8, 6	
	Triceps	6	3	10, 10, 8	
	Abdominal work	7	3	25, 25, 25	
	Forearm work	8	3	25, 25, 25	

Table 5.7d   Sample Power Phase Chart: Week 6

Day/week 6	Exercise	Station no.	No. of sets	Reps	% max.
Monday	Legs: core lift	1	3	8, 8, 6	See table 5.3.
	Legs: auxiliary	2	3	10, 10, 8	
	Shoulders: core	3	3	8, 8, 6	
	Shoulders: auxiliary	4	3	10, 10, 8	
	Legs: core lift	5	3	8, 8, 6	
	Shoulders: auxiliary	6	3	10, 10, 8	
	Forearm work	7	3	25, 25, 25	
	Abdominal work	8	3	25, 25, 25	
Wednesday	Chest: core lift	1	3	8, 8, 6	
	Chest: auxiliary	2	3	10, 10, 8	
	Biceps: core	3	3	8, 8, 6	
	Biceps: auxiliary	4	3	10, 10, 8	
	Abdominal work	5	3	25, 25, 25	
Friday	Back: core	1	3	8, 8, 6	
	Back: auxiliary	2	3	10, 10, 8	
	Triceps	3	3	10, 8, 6	
	Triceps	4	3	10, 8, 6	
	Back: core	5	3	8, 8, 6	
	Triceps	6	3	10, 10, 8	
	Abdominal work	7	3	25, 25, 25	
	Forearm work	8	3	25, 25, 25	

Table 5.7e   Sample Power Phase Chart: Week 7

Day/ week 7	Exercise	Station no.	No. of sets	Reps	% max.
Monday	Legs: core lift	1	3	8, 8, 6	See table 5.3.
	Legs: auxiliary	2	3	10, 10, 8	
	Shoulders: core	3	3	8, 6, 6	
	Shoulders: auxiliary	4	3	10, 10, 8	
	Legs: core lift	5	3	8, 6, 6	
	Shoulders: auxiliary	6	3	10, 10, 8	
	Forearm work	7	3	25, 25, 25	
	Abdominal work	8	3	25, 25, 25	
Wednesday	Chest: core lift	1	3	8, 6, 6	
	Chest: auxiliary	2	3	10, 10, 8	
	Biceps: core	3	3	8, 6, 6	
	Biceps: auxiliary	4	3	10, 10, 8	
	Abdominal work	5	3	25, 25, 25	
Friday	Back: core	1	3	8, 6, 6	
	Back: auxiliary	2	3	10, 10, 8	
	Triceps	3	3	10, 8, 6	
	Triceps	4	3	10, 8, 6	
	Back: core	5	3	8, 6, 6	
	Triceps	6	3	10, 10, 8	
	Abdominal work	7	3	25, 25, 25	
	Forearm work	8	3	25, 25, 25	

Specific Power Phase (Weeks 8-10)

Refer to table 5.8, a through c. This phase is designed to peak strength levels and gains. Because intensity levels are high, you need to pay proper attention to form and control. See table 5.5 for choice of exercises. Additional abdominal exercises can be found in chapter 9.

Table 5.8a Sample Specific Power Phase Chart: Week 8

Day/ week 8	Exercise	Station no.	No. of sets	Reps	% max.
Monday	Legs: core lift	1	3	6, 6, 4	See table 5.3.
	Legs: auxiliary	2	3	10, 10, 8	
	Shoulders: core	3	3	6, 6, 4	
	Shoulders: auxiliary	4	3	10, 10, 8	
	Legs: core lift	5	3	10, 10, 10	
	Shoulders: auxiliary	6	3	10, 10, 8	
	Forearm work	7	3	25, 25, 25	
	Abdominal work	8	3	6, 6, 4	
Wednesday	Chest: core lift	1	3	6, 6, 4	
	Chest: auxiliary	2	3	10, 10, 8	
	Biceps: core	3	3	10, 10, 8	
	Biceps: auxiliary	4	3	10, 10, 8	
	Abdominal work	5	3	10, 10, 8	
Friday	Back: core	1	3	10, 10, 8	
	Back: auxiliary	2	3	25, 25, 25	
	Triceps	3	3	10, 8, 6	
	Triceps	4	3	10, 10, 8	

(continued)

Table 5.8a   Sample Specific Power Phase Chart: Week 8   *(continued)*

Day/ week 8	Exercise	Station no.	No. of sets	Reps	% max.
Friday	Back: core	5	3	10, 8, 6	
	Triceps	6	3	10, 8, 6	
	Abdominal work	7	3	15, 12, 10	
	Forearm work	8	3	10, 10, 8	

Table 5.8b   Sample Specific Power Phase Chart: Week 9

Day/ week 9	Exercise	Station no.	No. of sets	Reps	% max.
Monday	Legs: core lift	1	3	6, 6, 4	See table 5.3.
	Legs: auxiliary	2	3	10, 10, 8	
	Shoulders: core	3	3	6, 6, 4	
	Shoulders: auxiliary	4	3	10, 10, 8	
	Legs: core lift	5	3	10, 10, 10	
	Shoulders: auxiliary	6	3	10, 10, 8	
	Forearm work	7	3	25, 25, 25	
	Abdominal work	8	3	6, 6, 4	
Wednesday	Chest: core lift	1	3	6, 6, 4	
	Chest: auxiliary	2	3	10, 10, 8	
	Biceps: core	3	3	10, 10, 8	
	Biceps: auxiliary	4	3	10, 10, 8	
	Abdominal work	5	3	10, 10, 8	

(continued)

Table 5.8b **Sample Specific Power Phase Chart:** **Week 9** *(continued)*

Day/ week 9	Exercise	Station no.	No. of sets	Reps	% max.
Friday	Back: core	1	3	10, 10, 8	
	Back: auxiliary	2	3	25, 25, 25	
	Triceps	3	3	10, 8, 6	
	Triceps	4	3	10, 10, 8	
	Back: core	5	3	10, 8, 6	
	Triceps	6	3	10, 8, 6	
	Abdominal work	7	3	15, 12, 10	
	Forearm work	8	3	10, 10, 8	
	Abdominal work	9	3	25, 25, 25	
	Forearm work	10	3	25, 25, 25	

Table 5.8c **Sample Specific Power Phase Chart:** **Week 10**

Day/ week 10	Exercise	Station no.	No. of sets	Reps	% max.
Monday	Legs: core lift	1	3	6, 4, 4	See table 5.3.
	Legs: auxiliary	2	3	10, 10, 8	
	Shoulders: core	3	3	6, 4, 4	
	Shoulders: auxiliary	4	3	10, 10, 8	
	Legs: core lift	5	3	6, 4, 4	
	Shoulders: auxiliary	6	3	10, 10, 8	
	Forearm work	7	3	25, 25, 25	
	Abdominal work	8	3	25, 25, 25	

(continued)

Table 5.8c   Sample Specific Power Phase Chart: Week 10   *(continued)*

Day/ week 10	Exercise	Station no.	No. of sets	Reps	% max.
Wednesday	Chest: core lift	1	3	6, 6, 4	
	Chest: auxiliary	2	3	10, 10, 8	
	Biceps: core	3	3	10, 10, 8	
	Biceps: auxiliary	4	3	10, 10, 8	
	Abdominal work	5	3	25, 25, 25	
Friday	Back: core	1	3	6, 6, 4	
	Back: auxiliary	2	3	25, 25, 25	
	Triceps	3	3	10, 8, 6	
	Triceps	4	3	10, 10, 8	
	Back: core	5	3	6, 6, 4	
	Triceps	6	3	10, 8, 6	
	Abdominal work	7	3	25, 25, 25	
	Forearm work	8	3	25, 25, 25	

Preseason Phase (Weeks 11-12)

Refer to table 5.9, a and b, and see table 5.5 for choice of exercises. See chapter 9 for additional abdominal exercises.

In-Season Strength Training

Because the in-season program involves combination training, which we have not discussed yet, we will provide sample workout charts for the in-season in chapter 11.

Table 5.9a   Sample Preseason Phase Chart: Week 11

Day/week 11	Exercise	Station no.	No. of sets	Reps	% max.
Monday	Bench press	1	3	10, 8, 6	See table 5.3.
	Pec dec	2	3	10, 10, 8	
	Squats	3	3	10, 8, 6	
	Leg curls	4	3	10, 10, 8	
	Bar dips	5	3	10, 10, 10	
	Abdominal work	6	3	10, 10, 8	
	Forearm work	7	3	25, 25, 25	
	Leg press	8	3	25, 25, 25	
Wednesday	Seated rows	1	3	10, 8, 6	
	One-arm rows	2	3	10, 10, 8	
	Preacher curls	3	3	10, 10, 8	
	Seated dumbbell curls	4	3	10, 10, 8	
	Lat pulldown	5	3	10, 10, 8	
	Hammer curls	6	3	10, 10, 8	
	Abdominal work	7	3	25, 25, 25	
Friday	Dumbbell military press	1	3	10, 8, 6	
	Side lateral raise	2	3	10, 10, 8	
	Triceps extension	3	3	10, 8, 6	
	Triceps kickbacks	4	3	10, 8, 6	
	Shrugs	5	3	15, 12, 10	
	Triceps pushdowns	6	3	10, 10, 8	
	Abdominal work	7	3	25, 25, 25	
	Forearm work	8	3	25, 25, 25	

Table 5.9b   Sample Preseason Phase Chart: Week 12

Day/ week 12	Exercise	Station no.	No. of sets	Reps	% max.
Monday	Bench press	1	3	10, 8, 6	See table 5.3.
	Pec dec	2	3	10, 10, 8	
	Squats	3	3	10, 8, 6	
	Leg curls	4	3	10, 10, 8	
	Bar dips	5	3	10, 10, 10	
	Abdominal work	6	3	10, 10, 8	
	Forearm work	7	3	25, 25, 25	
	Leg press	8	3	25, 25, 25	
Wednesday	Seated rows	1	3	10, 8, 6	
	One-arm rows	2	3	10, 10, 8	
	Preacher curls	3	3	10, 10, 8	
	Seated dumbbell curls	4	3	10, 10, 8	
	Lat pulldown	5	3	10, 10, 8	
	Hammer curls	6	3	10, 10, 8	
	Abdominal work	7	3	25, 25, 25	
Friday	Dumbbell military press	1	3	10, 8, 6	
	Side lateral raise	2	3	10, 10, 8	
	Triceps extension	3	3	10, 8, 6	
	Triceps kickbacks	4	3	10, 8, 6	
	Shrugs	5	3	15, 12, 10	
	Triceps pushdowns	6	3	10, 10, 8	
	Abdominal work	7	3	25, 25, 25	
	Forearm work	8	3	25, 25, 25	

CHAPTER 6

SPEED TRAINING

When we talk about increasing a

player's speed or agility, we have to do our homework. Do your players have the old five-page workout program that by the end of the year is so crumpled from being folded so many times that they can't even read what the exercises are anymore? We've experienced this even in professional baseball—handing out an eight-page work sheet for an entire season. Even then we knew there had to be more to increasing speed than that. So blindly we went off in search of a speed program designed specifically for baseball players. We wanted more than just the three-day-a-week-run-a-couple-of-miles-here-and-there program. We wanted something that was going to help us increase first-step explosion and help with reaction time. And we wanted to know how to link speed, power, and agility. In other words, we wanted the ultimate program.

Through trial, error, and persistence, we slowly started to put it together. We felt that if a strong emphasis on a skill such as taking hundreds of ground balls to the right side made us better fielders, then that same commitment was needed in a conditioning program. Now, we're not suggesting that you do hundreds of sprints at a time. What we're saying is that by improving your speed gradually, your training program will only help to enhance your baseball skills. And the key to gaining that half-step comes through the training and conditioning process. That original desire to take training to another level was the driving force for the program we've developed.

Before we describe our speed program, you should understand the role that speed plays in athletic performance. When you think of speed, you probably think of sprinting. But we all know that speed is much more involved than just merely being able to run or do some'hing quickly. Speed involves acceleration, which can begin from either a dead stop or from a cruising speed. To be fast, you must be able to accelerate or build speed quickly to reach your maximum or top speed. Simply put, speed is the maximum miles per hour that you can run, and acceleration is how quickly you reach that maximum. When we talk about improving speed, we're also talking about improving acceleration. When you possess speed, you rise above the average and make seemingly difficult maneuvers look easy. No matter how good your game already is, speed instantly raises it to another level and adds quality to your performance.

Contrary to popular opinion, we're all equipped with the necessary tools to run fast. That is, we can be taught to increase our speed. Given this information, we're making a mistake if we don't try to teach all our players to improve their speed.

SPEED COMPONENTS

Speed is basically a series of falls (or drives) and recoveries. The first movement, whether it be forward, backward, or lateral, involves falling. The degree the athlete falls is predetermined by the athlete and his technique. If he has been taught correct form, he'll likely be faster than the athlete with little or no running instruction. Improve the technique, and you automatically improve the fall, which leads to a quicker recovery step—and a faster athlete. The initial series of falls and recoveries is the acceleration phase. Once you're completely erect your fall and recovery series decreases in intensity and eventually your recovery steps become slower and longer. This is the maintenance phase. When determining the athlete's speed, we're really concentrating on lengthening and quickening this series of slow, long steps. In effect, stride length and stride frequency are the keys to speed.

$$\text{Speed} = \text{stride length} \times \text{stride frequency}$$

The technical process of a stride involves the drive phase and the recovery phase. The drive phase occurs when the foot applies force to the ground as it attempts to propel the body's center of gravity forward. It's easiest to understand this process if you picture a runner as he emerges from the starting blocks. He drives himself forward out of the blocks with as much power as he can to maximize his acceleration. The body lean or angle of a runner is determined by his leg strength and middle body strength. Because all force must go through the center of the body when running, strength in the abdominals and back is crucial. World-class sprinters effectively rehearse running mechanics beginning with the feet, extending to the ankle and knee, and then culminating at the gluteus. To improve speed, it's important to strengthen these muscle groups while improving stride mechanics.

The recovery phase of a stride occurs when the foot is off the ground. As the driving foot leaves the ground and begins the recovery phase, the heel is pulled back to the butt, creating the "kick back." The entire sprinting action requires the total coordination of the driving leg and the recovery leg in each of their phases. Once again, if we picture the sprinter coming out of the starting blocks, we can see that he is not only driving but recovering as well. The hip flexors, knees, and ankle joints are all working in combination to generate maximum angular velocity.

It is also important to focus on upper body alignment when teaching an athlete to run with proper form. The head, neck, and upper torso must be functioning as one moving part, and the eyes must be frozen, looking forward in their sockets. Moving the eyes around focuses the brain on different targets and interferes with the line of vision. You should not see the end of the distance until you've reached your peak acceleration. As you evolve from the acceleration to the maintenance phase, your body posture, if correct, should place your line of vision at the destination. Your only effort now should be to maintain your peak speed.

We don't want to forget about the importance of the arms in determining how fast an athlete will run. The arms counterbalance the stride action, resulting in an opposite arm–opposite leg relationship. The hands should be slightly open and extend backward to the hip or slightly behind it and forward to the height of the shoulder so that the bottom joint of the thumb does not rise above the shoulder. The biceps, forearms,

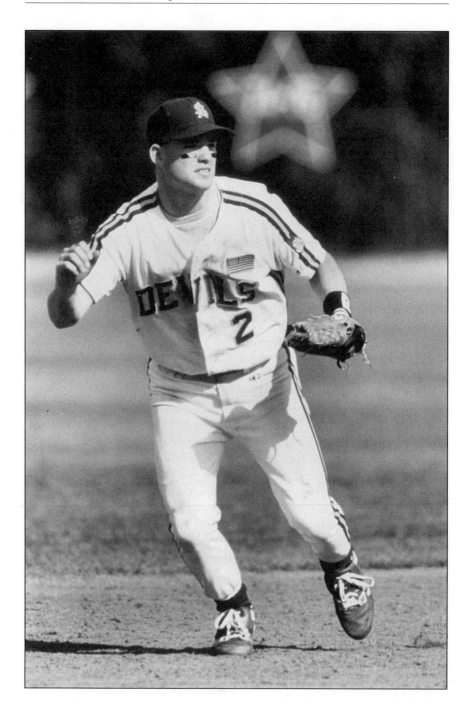

and wrists must be strong since the arm drive down and back will determine the extent of the forward or backward movement. The quicker you pump your arms in a backward and forward motion, the quicker the strides will turn over, and the faster you will run.

BASEBALL-SPECIFIC SPEED

How do the speed phases (acceleration and maintenance) and stride phases (drive and recovery) relate to baseball players? For one, while playing on defense ballplayers must drive and recover laterally, backward and forward. As they switch to offense, they must run straight or linearly down the base path while running on a curve around the bases. Base runners use great acceleration and speed between the bases, especially considering that the distance to pick up speed is greatly reduced by base leads and slide zones.

As base runners, baseball players are unique in that while attempting to steal bases they must run in one direction while looking another. As he attempts to steal second base, for example, a player must fall toward second base while looking toward home plate. The player benefits by being able to add to the intensity and recovery of the fall by looking inside. It also helps him to locate the ball and determine his course of action such as sliding into second, or rounding second and continuing to third should the catcher mishandle the ball. On defense, the same applies for infielders and outfielders as they handle ground balls and track fly balls.

When playing defense, baseball players often need the ability to run backward effectively as well as forward. The same principles that apply to running fast forward are used to run fast backward. The upper torso, neck, and back alignment and the brain's line of vision are still key factors, with the main difference being the upper torso posture. While the athlete running forward has a leaning posture, the athlete running backward has a more upright posture. Again, arm swing and arm stride coordination are as crucial for backward speed as they are for forward speed.

IMPROVING YOUR SPEED

Now that we know what speed is and how it applies to baseball, let's take a look at what we can do to improve speed. There are four primary methods to employ when developing speed:

1. Strength training
2. Plyometric exercises
3. Traditional sprint-training techniques
4. Sprint-assisted methods

These methods can be further categorized by calling weight training, plyometric exercises, and traditional sprint-training techniques resisted speed-training methods. Basically this means that all of these exercises and drills work to improve the *stride length*. Sprint-assisted methods fall into their own category of assisted speed training that target the *stride frequency*.

Now if we go back to the basic premise that speed is the product of stride length and stride frequency, we'll see that strength and power in our legs are the key factors to increasing stride length. And the stronger and more powerful our arms and torso become, the faster we are able to pump our arms, which in turn leads to increased stride frequency. Overall body strength and power therefore are crucial for improving your speed. And one of the most effective ways of improving your overall body strength and power is through strength training.

Power—the rate at which work is performed—is essential to moving faster. The more powerful the muscle fiber activated at the time of explosion, the more force is exerted on the ground, and the faster you go. Given enough time, any person who could run could perform a 40-yard dash. However, we want our athletes to perform this sprint with power and speed. An elephant is very powerful and also very slow moving, while a cheetah creates tremendous power from extraordinary speed.

The main focus of our weight-training program for speed is on the large muscles used in sprinting: the gluteus maximus, quadriceps, hamstrings, and calves. The secondary focus is on the arms, chest, back, and abdominals. Again, remember that weight training falls into the category of resisted speed training, our goal being to increase stride length.

The second form of resisted training is plyometric exercises, which are covered more extensively in chapter 8. These exercises help improve speed by focusing on the explosive movement necessary for increasing speed. Plyometrics are explosive exercises requiring a great deal of strength that teach the nervous system to fire faster, which in turn results in faster movement. These exercises also help develop good coordination and agility.

Traditional sprint-training techniques round out the resisted speed training methods. Typically, these techniques include flexibility, proper running form, uphill sprinting, starting techniques, speed endurance, and movement patterns specific to baseball. Because these are the more traditional methods, you may be familiar with most of them and how they work. Some of these traditional methods include running sprints, incorporating ladders and hurdles, and running hills, all of which we've probably done at one time or another. These methods are considered traditional simply because they've been around a long time and are widely used at all levels of the game. We have included a hurdle drill, but for the most part we focus on some of the newer techniques.

The assisted training methods of speed training include towing training, treadmill training, and downhill running. Recall that the main goal of assisted training methods is to increase your stride frequency. Also included in assisted training methods are overspeed drills, which force the body to move faster than its normal top speed. This type of training causes your nerves to contract faster than normal and trains your body to overcome rejections of faster movement. It helps retrain your neuromuscular coordination to work faster; used regularly, these drills will eventually lead to improved stride frequency, longer strides, and a longer top speed with a more relaxed and controlled running form.

RESISTED SPEED DRILLS

ARM SWING

Focus: The mechanical arm swing involved during running

Procedure:

1. Start with your shoulders in a tall upright position and your head in fixed position.

2. Keep your arms in a 90-degree angle but not tightly locked.

3. Bring your hands up to an imaginary line at your jaw and back to a point where your hand touches your pocket. Your arm action should be quick like a piston but not stiff.

Duration: 10 to 15 reps with each arm or timed intervals of 10 to 12 seconds

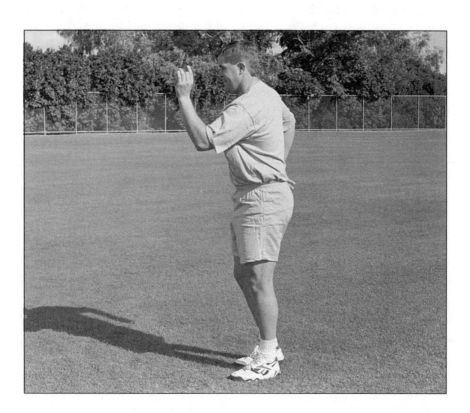

STEP-UPS

Focus: The leg drive and arm swing involved during running; gluteals, hamstrings, quadriceps

Procedure:

1.   Start with your right leg securely planted on a box and your left leg on the ground.

2.   Your arm should be cocked in running position form with your left arm in the upswing position to create opposite arm-opposite leg action.

3.   Drive your left leg and right arm up simultaneously. Keep proper running form—toe up, heel up, knee up—during the leg drive.

4.   Return your leg to the ground and repeat immediately to create a firing pattern with the leg and arm drive.

Duration: 10 to 15 reps on each leg or timed intervals of 10 to 12 seconds for each leg

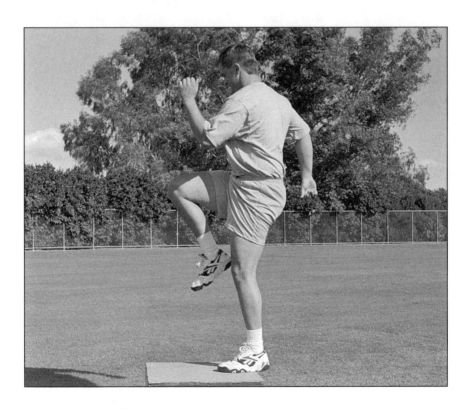

LEG LIFTS OVER MINI-HURDLES

Focus: The mechanics of running with proper leg lift and arm swing; entire leg and calf region

Procedure:

1.   Line up 12-inch high "hurdles" about 1 1/2 yards apart.
2.   Start with a light run up to hurdles.
3.   With proper sprinting mechanics and aggressive arm swing and leg lift, take two strides between each hurdle.

Repetitions: 4 to 6 per set, 3 to 4 sets.

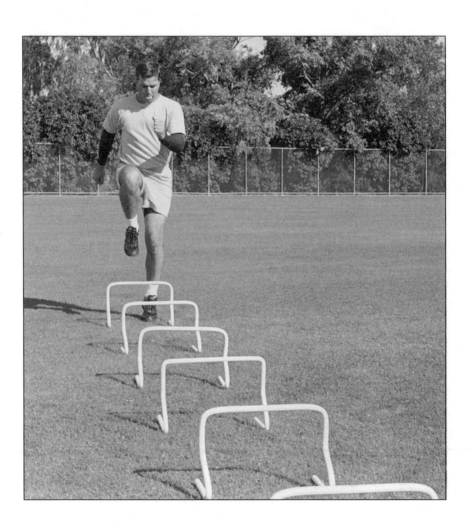

VELOCITY BUILDER ARM KICKS

Focus: Range of motion of hamstrings and gluteals; the aggressive leg swing from the gluteal area involved in running

Procedure:

1. Start with your arms extended in front of your body at about shoulder level.

2. In an alternating fashion with your leg straight (slight bend in knee), kick your right leg up to your right hand and your left leg up to your left hand.

Repetitions: 10 to 15 with each leg, 3 to 4 sets

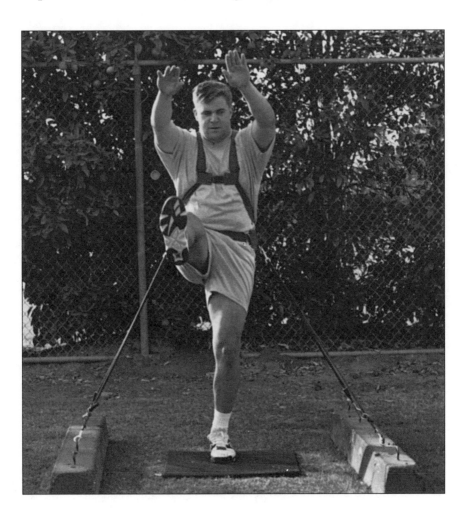

VELOCITY BUILDER KNEE-TO-SHOULDER LIFTS

Focus: The aggressive knee lift and drive force created when running; muscle hip flexors, gluteals, hamstring, quadriceps

Procedure:

1.   Place your hands between your legs to avoid excess upper body movement and keep your arms out of the way. With an explosive skipping action, drive your right knee toward your right shoulder.

2.   Focus on proper leg lift technique.

3.   Keep your torso upright for full range of motion.

Repetitions: 10 to 15 with each leg, 3 to 4 sets

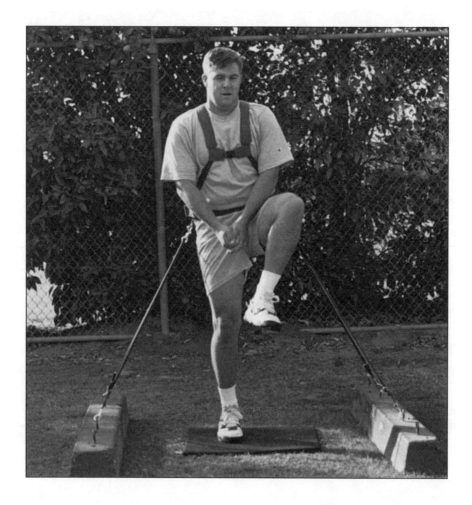

MEDICINE BALL TOSS WITH A BASE STEAL SPRINT

Focus: Explosive stage of the crossover step involved in stealing a base

Procedure:

1. Start in a base-stealing position.

2. In a hip toss fashion, explosively throw a medicine ball across your body. The momentum will create an overspeed effect that will make your jumps more explosive.

3. Run the medicine ball down before it stops rolling and repeat.

Repetitions: Five 10- to 15-yard tosses per set, 3 to 4 sets

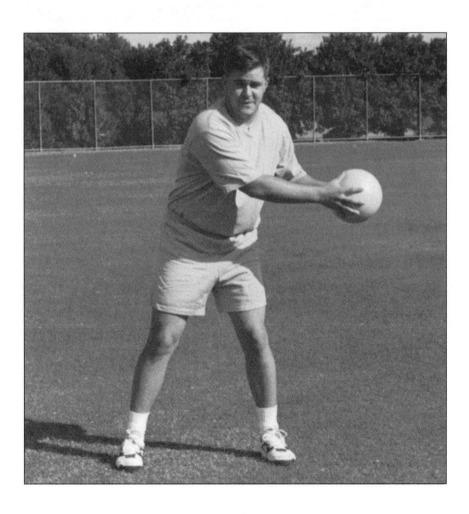

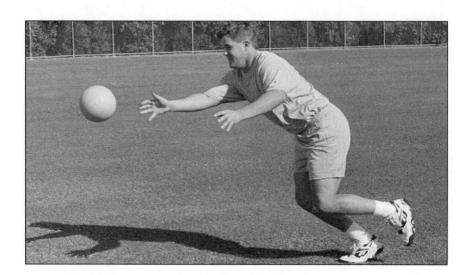

SLED TOWS

Focus: Acceleration phase of the sprint; explosive starts

Procedure:

1. With a speed harness or belt securely fastened to a sled, tow the sled 10 to 20 yards.

2. Release the sled and immediately sprint for 20 yards. Sled can also be used for backpedaling.

3. Use 10 to 20 percent of your body weight for the sled. Do not exceed 20 percent of body weight.

Repetitions: Two pulls of 20 yards per set, 2 to 3 sets.

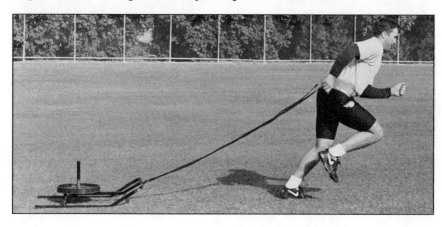

ASSISTED SPEED DRILLS

ACCELERATIONS

Focus: The initial build of force during the first 5 yards of a sprint; leg and hip muscles, gluteals, and upper body muscles

Procedure:

1. Using a speed belt harness, towel, or tow rope, a partner applies moderate resistance while runner runs at maximum speed, pulling the partner.

2. Practice good body lean and good running mechanics.

Repetitions: Start with five tows of 10 yards each, eventually building up to maximum of 20-yard tows

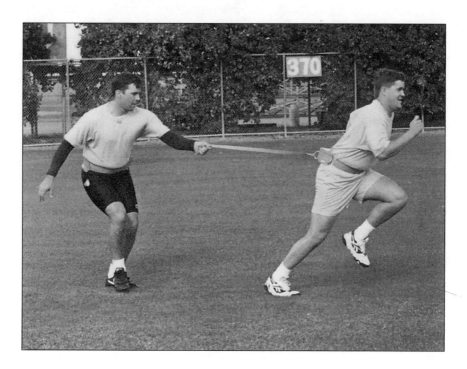

BREAKAWAY TOWS

Focus: Acceleration phase of the sprint

Procedure:

1. Using a speed belt harness, towel, or tow rope, a partner applies moderate medium resistance to the runner for 5 yards.

2. Release the resistance and runner sprints for 15 more yards.

3. When the resistance is released, runner should feel the freedom of explosive acceleration. This is what we're teaching the body to get a feel for.

Repetitions: 5 to 8 sprints

Repetitions: Two pulls of 20 yards per set, 2 to 3 sets.

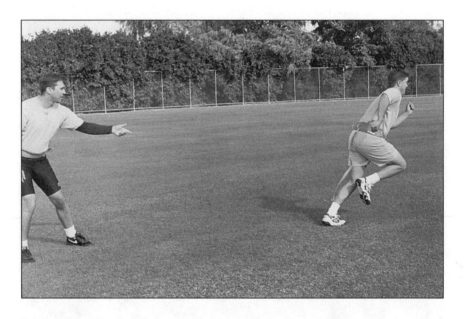

OVERSPEED/RESISTANCE BOUNDS

Focus: Explosive drive phase of the arm swing and leg lift

Procedure:

1. With resistance applied by partner, tow rope, or properly moni-
    tored and supervised flexicord, bound out the same as a deer
    bounds out.

2. Use proper running mechanics and, to increase stride length, focus
    on gaining as much distance as you can with your stride.

Repetitions: 10- to 20-yard bounds with 4 to 5 per set, 3 to 4 sets

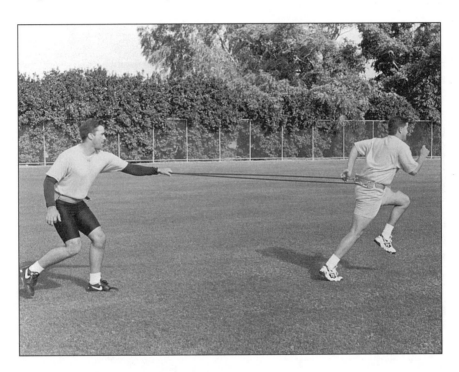

BOUNDS WITH OVERSPEED

Focus: The overspeed component of sprint training; teaching the body to run faster

Procedure:

1.   With tow cord or flexicord properly attached in overspeed fashion, runner is pulled.

2.   Gain as much ground as possible. With overspeed training, the runner focuses on staying relaxed and in a controlled overspeed process.

3.   Also helps to teach the body to maintain top speeds longer.

Repetitions: 10- to 20-yard bounds with 4 to 5 per set, 3 to 4 sets

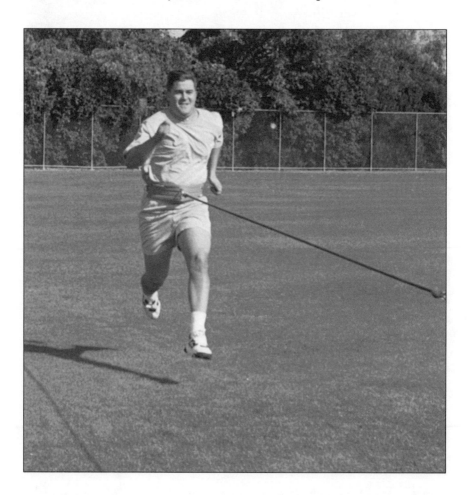

GET-UP SPRINTS

Focus: Overspeed component of the sprint

Procedure:

1. With flexicord stretched to its safest maximum length, on command get up from a seated position and explode into a good running position.

2. This drill adds an element of reaction and explosive acceleration.

Variations: Also try this drill from kneeling or lying down.

Repetitions: Three to four 20-yard sprints per set, 3 to 4 sets

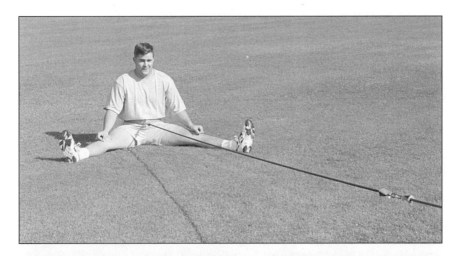

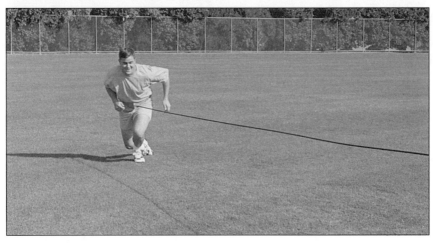

CHAPTER 7

AGILITY TRAINING

Speed development for baseball

players would not be complete if we didn't also include a section on improving agility. After all, the outstanding plays you see in the field are often a result of speed combined with agility. So, what exactly is agility? We'll define it here as the body's ability to change direction while maintaining its speed.

The key to improving agility is to minimize the loss of speed when shifting your body's center of gravity. Drills that require rapid changes of direction forward, backward, laterally, and vertically will help you improve your agility as well as your coordination by training your body to make these changes in movement more quickly. Once you've mastered the agility drills in this chapter, you can then increase your coordination development by adding ball-handling skills along with the applicable footwork drills we've included in this chapter. And coordination—the ability to synchronize all aspects of athleticism—is the basis for any successful athlete, regardless of the sport.

Diamond sport athletes are involved primarily in quick, explosive movements. Lateral speed, agility, and quickness are often just as important as strength and speed. Baseball requires players to position in various angles ranging from straight up to bent over. They need to be able to react with quickness, strength, and explosion from any of these angles. Explosion out of the box, the thrust when stealing a base, and the charge off the mound to field a bunt after a pitch are all examples of explosive movements with your body in an opposite direction. When working to build explosion and agility, we must work with a systematic training approach specific to our individual sport's needs. Ideally, we'd like our players to move like Ken Griffey, Jr., on the fly or Alex Rodriguez in the hole. Our workouts aim to condition the body and incorporate fun and variety while obtaining maximum gains in agility.

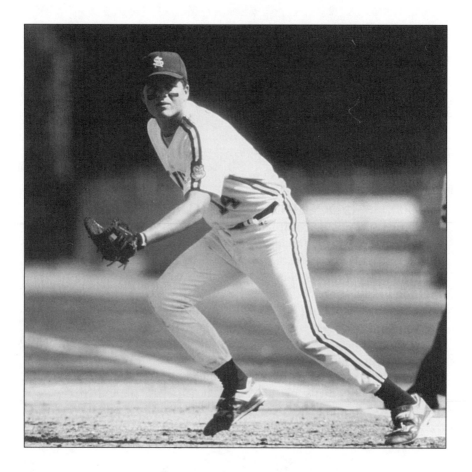

AGILITY TRAINING OBJECTIVES

By setting goals to challenge yourself to add to the intensity and master the movement, and by consistently concentrating on the details of your workout, you'll see improvements in your baseball-specific agility. Here are the objectives of our agility drills:

1. To increase intramuscular coordination. The drills aim to teach your muscles and your body to perform specific baseball movements at a high speed.

2. To develop more explosive power, speed, and strength of the major muscle groups. To get the most explosive power from your body, you need adequate strength in the large muscle groups.

3. To make quickness a habit. Training at maximum firing efforts teaches muscles and feet to fire more quickly.

EDUCATING YOUR BODY FOR AGILITY

Agility consists of many independent parts involving the eyes, brain, muscles, and coordination. Four main phases of agility are

1. *Recognition*—what your eyes see,

2. *Reaction*—explosion with your body,

3. *Reach*—forceful thrust that propels you at an efficient angle, and

4. *Recovery*—your ability to balance and regather quickly.

The first stage is recognition. This is when you first see the event that triggers your reaction. For instance, when fielding, it's the moment you see the ball hit and heading your way. You react by adjusting your position to place yourself in the best spot to field the ball. You may need to reach to make the catch and then recover to throw the ball in. How quickly and accurately you go through these four stages depends on your level of agility.

Quick movements result from ballistic firing patterns within the neuromuscular system that signal the muscle fibers to react. Genetics play a key role in the ratio of fast-twitch to slow-twitch muscle fibers an individual possesses, and this ratio cannot be changed. However, training can selectively increase the size of each type of muscle fiber. In explosive, quick movements, fast-twitch muscle fibers are the predominant muscle fibers recruited to action. Thus, by repeatedly training these fibers through explosive action drills, you'll not only sharpen the neuromuscular pathways necessary for the quick movement, you'll also enlarge the size of the involved fast-twitch fibers.

We can increase quickness and agility only by increasing the firing rate of the neuromuscular system. That is, we must train our feet and arms to move faster. Training our systems to perform at maximum speed is the only way to achieve our quickness and agility goals. For instance, we must teach our feet to apply a greater force when they impact the ground. The lighter the impact, the greater the force, and this can only be achieved with rapid movement of the feet. Combining this increase in quickness with a change in direction is how we improve agility. Many of the movements are similar in increasing speed or agility, but the key difference is the added change of direction either laterally, vertically, forward, or backward.

POWER FOR AGILITY

To move faster in baseball, you must gain power. You need to activate your large muscles quickly and explosively to transfer power to competitive speed and quickness for baseball. Focus your power work on your power zone. The leg muscles, midsection, and gluteals do the majority of work. Here's a breakdown of the power zone where the major focus of muscle strength should be placed for maximum gains in agility:

• The drive muscles—hamstrings, quadriceps, gluteals—supply tremendous power, but you have to use their strength. You must challenge and teach these muscles to rapidly fire for short periods of time. Explosions in various directions and angles are necessary to simulate game situations as much as possible.

• The hip and lateral muscles—hip flexors, adductors, abductors—play a major role in lateral movement, change of direction, and crossover steps. Challenge these muscles with drills and strength training to give them the ability to perform these movements with tremendous quickness.

• Torso muscles—abdominals, lower back—are perhaps the most important components of lateral quickness. Motion is initiated through the torso. If this area is weak and neglected, the torso reacts slowly to messages sent from the central nervous system. Baseball is a rotational sport, which means we're often moving left and right with our upper torso while our legs remain fixed or moving in a constant direction. As a result, strong abdominals and a strong lower back are essential.

Powerful, quick, explosive movements coupled with change of direction require whole body development. Focus on working the power zone or core section of the body. The explosive nature you need must come from the education of high-speed output.

Enhanced agility and coordination not only improve athletic performance but also help reduce the risk of injury. Many players avoid injury as they dive or roll by being agile and coordinated and knowing where they are in relation to the ground, fence, base, and other players. Agility and coordination allow them to take an impact with a minimum of stress to their bodies. Of course not all injuries can be avoided, but the well-conditioned player will always recover more quickly and with less strain than the player who is not as highly conditioned.

AGILITY DRILLS

These drills for improving agility and coordination may be unfamiliar to you, but they are drills through which even beginners will benefit. As you learn these exercises and drills better, focus on the finer points of each drill and then add ball-handling skills.

The first four of the following agility drills are performed on the side kick box, a powerful neuromuscular plyometric training tool that incorporates power from the push-off force of the angled box. The side kick enhances and teaches good foot speed and agility from the forceful and rhythmic tapping of the feet.

REACH RUNS

Focus: Calf area; the explosive action of pushing off the balls of the feet to create quick feet

Procedure:

1.   The run rhythm is 1, 2, up; 1, 2, up. Push up and off explosively, pulling your toe, heel, and knee up as you do when you're running.

2.   Perform all movements quickly in short bursts of 10 to 15 seconds. This will teach your feet to move faster.

3.   Start the movement slowly until you get the feel and balance required, then increase speed.

Duration: 10 to 15 seconds or 3 per set, 3 to 4 sets

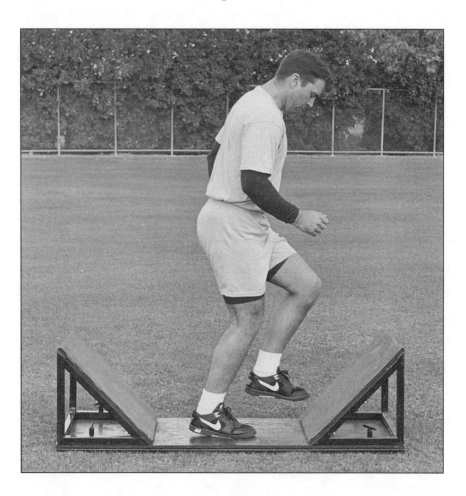

BACK REACH RUNS

Focus: Calf area; the explosive action of pushing off the balls of the feet to create quick feet

Procedure:

1. The run rhythm is 1, 2, up; 1, 2, up. Push up and off explosively, reaching backward.

2. Perform all movements quickly in short bursts of 10 to 15 seconds.

3. Start the movement slowly until you get the feel and balance required, then increase speed.

Duration: 10 to 15 seconds or 3 per set, 3 to 4 sets

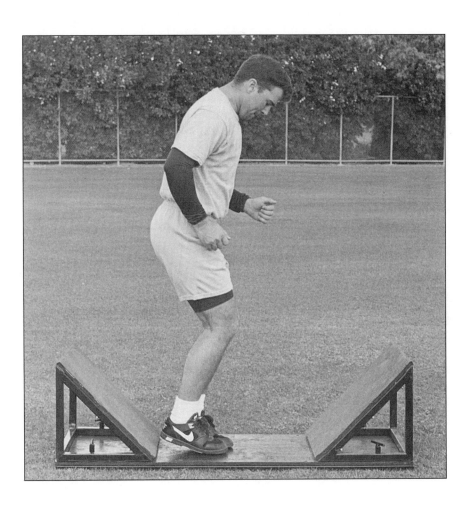

SIDE-SHUFFLE

Focus: Calves, legs, hips

Procedure:

1. The run rhythm is 1, 2, up; 1, 2, up. Begin facing sideways in the center of the platform. Extend your right leg out and push up and off the angle board explosively. The force and momentum of the push will push you back to the center, where you will get the 1, 2 rhythm. Then repeat on the opposite side.

2. Perform all movements quickly in short bursts of 10 to 15 seconds. This will help teach your feet to move faster.

3. Start the movement slowly until you get the feel and balance required, then increase speed.

Duration: 10 to 15 seconds or 3 per set, 3 to 4 sets

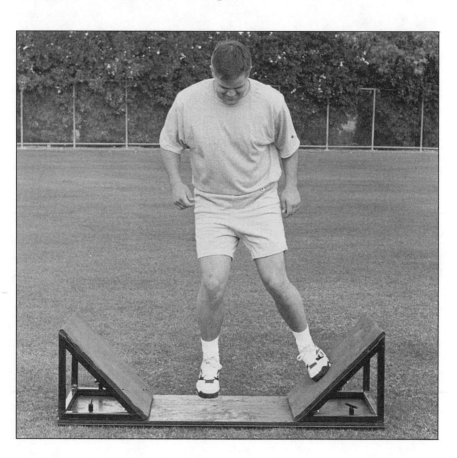

CROSSOVER

Focus: Calves, legs, hips

Procedure:

1. The rhythm is 1, 2, up; 1, 2, up. This exercise is similar to side-shuffles except that you'll cross one leg over the other to push off of the angle board and then repeat the procedure on the opposite side.

2. Perform all movements quickly in short bursts of 10 to 15 seconds.

3. Start the movement slowly until you get the feel and balance required, then increase speed.

Duration: 10 to 15 seconds or 3 per set, 3 to 4 sets

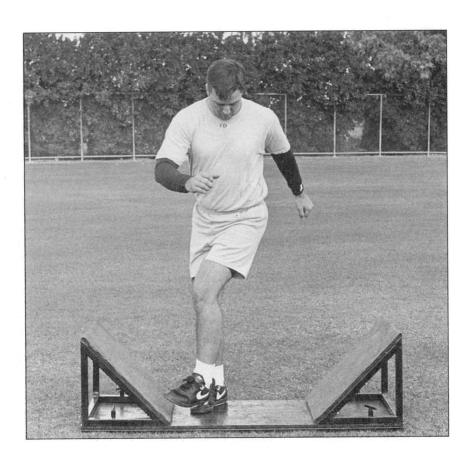

LATERAL HIGH KNEES

Focus: Explosive change of direction

Procedure:

1.   Move laterally in a running motion across mini-hurdles, working on lifting your knees and pumping your arms quickly and explosively.

2.   Change direction at the end and come back in the same manner.

Duration: 10 to 15 seconds or 3 per set, 3 to 4 sets

LATERAL HIGH KNEES WITH RESISTANCE

Focus: Overspeed resistance

Procedure:

1.   Wearing a resistance cord and belt attached to a fixed object or held stationary by a partner, move laterally in a running motion across hurdles, working on lifting knees and pumping arms quickly and explosively.

2.   Change direction at the end and come back in the same manner.

Duration: 10 to 15 seconds or 3 per set, 3 to 4 sets

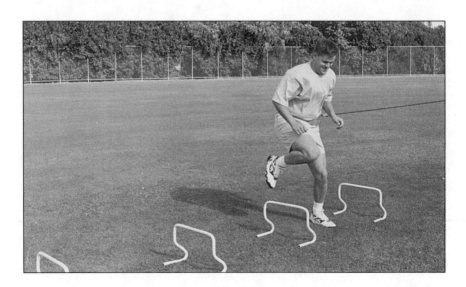

LATERAL BOX RUNS

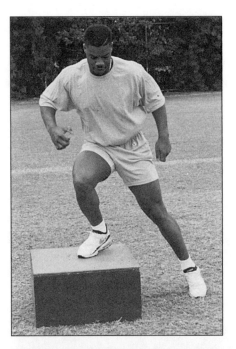

Focus: Explosive lateral movement in the hip flexors and entire leg region

Procedure:

1. On a 12-inch plyometric box, start with your right leg or left leg slightly bent on the box and the other leg slightly bent on the ground.

2. Simultaneously and rhythmically pump your arms and push with both legs in an alternating fashion.

3. Stay light and quick with your feet as you touch the ground and the box.

Duration: 10 to 15 second intervals, 3 to 4 sets

SLIDE BOARD

Focus: Explosive quadriceps, hamstrings, and gluteals

Procedure:

1. Start in an upright position with a soft bend in your knees.
2. Go into a slight squat and swing your right leg behind you in a speed-skating fashion.
3. Push off the side support and glide to the other side immediately.
4. When you touch the opposite side, return and continue movement.

Duration: 10- to 15-second intervals or 3 per set, 3 to 4 sets

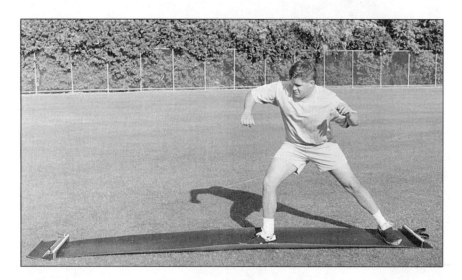

CHAPTER 8

PLYOMETRIC TRAINING

The pitcher winds up, here's the

pitch, it's a fastball for a strike on the outside corner—excellent pitch that registered 90 mph on the radar gun. . . . Okay, here comes the pitch, the batter swings—oh my! What a tremendous drive to the upper deck! . . . Gwynn hits a liner to right field, he rounds second, the outfielder throws home, it's going to be close, here he comes—he's out! . . . The pitcher comes set, the base runner leads off first, here's the pitch, and the base runner breaks with an outstanding jump and—he's safe at second base!

These are plays we've all seen at baseball games. The description of the plays would be announced just as we listed them—short bursts of explosive movements by pitchers, catchers, outfielders, batters, and base runners. It is these explosive baseball-specific movements—often performed at or near 100 percent maximum efforts—that plyometric training sharpens.

WHAT ARE PLYOMETRICS?

Plyometric exercises may be new to you, but they have been around for some time. The Soviets pioneered the use of plyometric exercises back in the mid 1960s, and their effectiveness was evident in the Soviets' virtual monopoly of sprinting and track and field events during the 1960s and 1970s. Not until the 1980s did the sporting community in general begin to realize the potential gains from the use of these training techniques.

In plyometric training the muscles and their elastic components are rapidly stretched when landing from a jump and immediately follow that landing with another rapid and powerful jump or hop in a vertical or horizontal direction. This stretching of the muscle's elastic components produces a rubber band-like effect in the connective tissue as it snaps back from the initial stretch. A stretch reflex is also initiated when landing, which leads the stretched muscle to contract forcefully and eventually provides greater force for a longer or higher jump or bound. This series of bounding and jumping exercises is one of the best ways to develop explosive force.

TRAINING THE MUSCLES TO REACT

Plyometrics bridge the gap between speed and strength to create a force known as power. A muscle's ability to react forcefully and quickly requires the muscle system to switch rapidly from eccentric (negative) contractions to concentric (positive) contractions. This reaction of the muscles is possible because of a reflex response within each muscle called the stretch or myotatic reflex response. The greater the stretch put on the resting muscle length prior to the concentric contraction, the greater load the muscle can lift or force it can exert. This force is often referred to as explosive power. The actual rate of the stretch is more significant than its size. And because this reflex response occurs in all phases of baseball, many major league teams have incorporated some type of plyometric training into their conditioning programs. Let's look at an example to help give us a better idea of the myotatic reflex response process.

When an infielder steps up to his ready position he sends a message to his muscles to go on alert because something is getting ready to happen. The message is urgent because the athlete is in competition and will need to move rapidly and explosively in some direction when the bat meets the ball. The process of preparing for this move is the myotatic reflex response. Its next component is a stimuli to make the muscle fire. The stimuli of the response obviously is where the baseball goes. This process occurs so quickly that it is basically a neuromuscular response or an interaction between muscles and nerves except that it works in conjunction with the rapid muscle contractions known as the myotatic reflex response. Since baseball is a game where players are constantly reacting to stimuli, it makes sense that we would want to enhance the body's ability to react quickly.

Basically, plyometric training helps develop the nervous system so it will respond with maximal reactive force. Through plyometric training, the eccentric and concentric contraction process is taught to occur more rapidly and forcefully. This helps us to move quicker in the field, react more forcefully at the plate, and deliver more velocity when we throw the baseball. If you have any doubts about the advantages of plyometric training, ask Cleveland's Matt Williams for his opinion. His game has benefited immeasurably from a routine plyometric training program.

The concept of plyometrics is often misunderstood and misapplied in training programs. Enhancing the speed of the contraction in the muscle and increasing the force with that added speed is the goal of plyometric training. This is the bridge that turns strength gains in the weight room into functional baseball speed and movements.

Here's what occurs during plyometrics and how this training helps to enhance our explosive power:

- Plyometrics is the linking of speed and strength for the development of reactive power.

- It incorporates an eccentric and concentric contraction coming together. Where the two meet there is housed energy or, simply put, power. The quicker you can overcome an eccentric movement with a concentric movement, the more explosive you can be.

- It places load on muscles, and when a muscle is stretched too much, the myotatic reflex response is initiated to keep the muscle from overstretching and to make the contraction change direction. By combining the two—the load and the reflex response—power is produced. This is a split-second response.

- It teaches and helps to develop good coordination and agility.

- It helps to develop the explosive strength needed in speed, lateral movement, and acceleration.

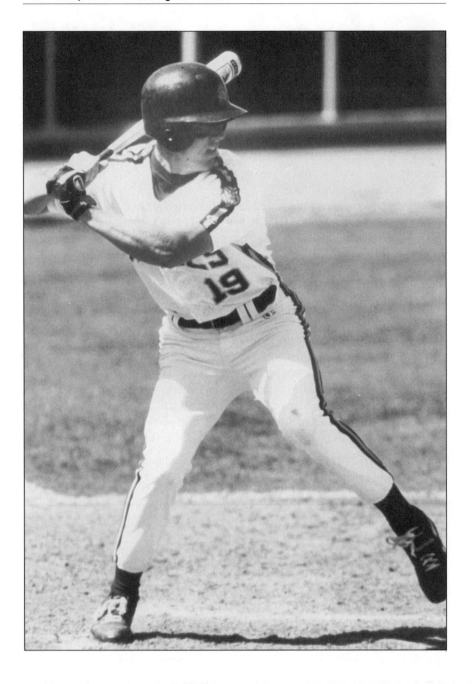

Assuring the Necessary Strength Base

For the best results, do plyometrics along with a good strength program, as plyometric training alone is not enough to build the power-speed combination. Building a proper strength base in the muscles, tendons, ligaments, cartilage, and bone will decrease the chances of injury from the high amounts of stress plyometrics place on the body. Strength also gives us more potential force we can apply. The more force, the greater our chances of increasing the speed of a movement, thus giving us more power.

Improving the Rate of Muscle Stretch

To get the most out of plyometric training, the exercises should be done with maximum intensity and quickness. The rate or how quickly the muscle stretches has a greater impact on power gains than how far they are stretched. This simply means that the number of repeated jumps are not as important as the intensity and speed at which they are performed. Fatigue sets in rapidly with successive jumps, and fatigue limits the reactive ability of the nervous system. Remember that we are training to create maximum force in the shortest amount of time that we can. This takes us back to the principle that the quicker a muscle stretches, the greater its impact is in applying force or power.

We know the reactive ability is when the muscle system switches from the eccentric phase to the concentric phase. If the force required to stop this process takes too long to switch from one phase to the other, the benefits are lost. For example, when jumping off of a box, we want to spend minimal time on the ground. We want to redirect the force that brought us down from the box back up or out as quickly as possible. Our goal here is to react as quickly as we can with the greatest force that we can. This is also how we train the nervous system to react and respond quickly. Baseball is an explosive reactive sport, so we must train in this way.

Plyometrics should only be performed when a player can do them quickly and at a high intensity. If you perform plyometrics any other way, you're actually teaching the neuromuscular system to perform at a slower rate instead of at the quick-fire rate needed in baseball. Coaches should allow proper rest intervals between sets so that players can perform at maximum intensity.

Increasing Applied Force

When we're looking at standard limitations for players, how can we get them to go beyond these limitations or train their bodies with a greater amount of force than they can or will produce? When Joe Carter blasts a tape measure shot of 450 feet plus, he seems to defy human capabilities in strength measurements. If we look at the law of physics, his feat is almost a mathematical impossibility. As baseball fans and enthusiasts, we see it happen often. You might say these are gifted and skilled athletes, and I would have to agree. So I raise the question, "Why then could a power lifter with tremendous strength not match this feat even if he took his 100 best cuts?" Seventy-five percent of his chances we could chalk up to his lack of experience and skill in baseball. However, the remaining 25 percent are likely due to his neuromuscular system not being adapted to the quick-fire response he needs to hit a baseball with maximum force. The split-second link of speed and strength occurs often when we perform in baseball. We practice the skill movements daily so our body is more adapted to the responses it takes to make this possible.

How, then, do we get the body to perform beyond prescribed limits? Mother Nature is our biggest aid. Gravity helps us to produce greater amounts of force. For example, if you were to drop a baseball onto Mike Piazza's head from six inches, the impact would be minimal. Now, drop the baseball from six feet. Obviously, Mike would feel considerably more impact and may become upset! It's gravity that increases the force with which the baseball strikes.

When gravity is applied to a player's body when he is performing plyometrics, the forces elicited are tremendous. If a 220-pound player jumps off a four-foot box, he'll load his muscles with force greater than a ton. To be precise, during this brief instant his nervous system recruits enough fibers to stop and redirect 2,489 pounds of force. Coming off a four-foot box, his muscles are contracting at the rate it takes to jump 48 inches. Simply put, with plyometric training, he can apply more force than his body could ever possibly do alone. These forces can be increased by combining plyometrics with a strength and power program. With power a big part of the game, plyometrics is a great way to train to enhance this area.

PLYOMETRIC SAFETY AND TECHNIQUE

Jumping exercises place a high demand on the hip, knee, and ankle joints, tendons, muscles, and the neuromuscular system, so they must be learned well and performed correctly. Consider a player's age and physical and skill development before starting him on a plyometric

Injury Prevention Tips

1. Have a proper warm-up. Make sure muscles are properly warmed for at least 5 to 10 minutes and ready for explosive movements.
2. Wear proper foot wear. Wear shoes with good ankle support and stability.
3. Exercise on a firm but giving surface such as grass, turf, or a track.
4. Use a sturdy padded box with a solid base.
5. Use proper progression. Start slow and progress moderately.
6. Consider any special circumstances as well as the player's age, size, ability, and body structure.

Proper Mechanics

1. Swing your arms from the shoulders to help thrust yourself forward or upward.
2. Make sure your middle body is upright and straight from your hips to your head.
3. Land properly, flexing at the knees, ankles, and hips to absorb impact.
4. Take proper rest periods so your energy system can replenish itself.

program. Advanced or stringent plyometrics should be prohibited for children under 14 because of possible injury to the spine and lower body joints. Monitor the load of exercises carefully and allow for proper recovery time between sets.

Again, proper technique is vital when performing plyometric exercises. Make sure correct posture is taught and adhered to. Shoulders should be squared and the torso should always be in an upright position with abdominals tight to avoid back injury. Knees should always be bent when jumping and landing and the butt tucked underneath the hips and back. Balance is important in these exercises. Before advancing to highly skilled movements, make sure you and your players know the basics. All take-offs should be explosive. Upon ground impact, the hip, knees, and ankles should be fully flexed to achieve good balance and coordination.

Plyometrics will greatly enhance any training program, but these exercises need to be monitored. Teach proper mechanics and incorporate various exercises and programs. Have fun and be creative. Teach your players to enjoy making themselves better.

RAPID BOX JUMPS

Focus: Building explosive power in the entire calf and quadriceps area

Procedure:

1. Start on the ground in front of a plyometric box.
2. Bend your knees and lower your butt slightly.
3. Explosively but with control jump up on box, then jump down.
4. When your feet hit the ground, immediately jump back on the box. Spend as little time as you can on the ground.

Variations: The jumps can be done with varying box heights as players build up the needed strength. (This can be determined by their ability to perform the jumps at the required height with the suggested number of repetitions.)

Repetitions: 6 to 10, 2 to 3 sets

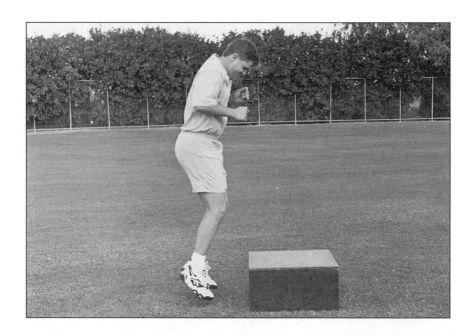

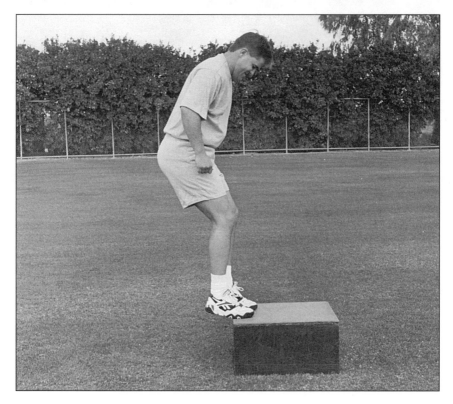

ALTERNATING HEIGHT BOX JUMPS

Focus: Quadriceps, hamstrings, gluteals, calf muscles

Procedure:

1. Use three to five plyometric boxes of various heights from 12 to 24 inches, placed in a straight line about two feet apart.

2. Starting with the smallest box first, perform box jumps box to box.

3. Spend as little time on the ground as possible. Various heights will help to develop explosive power.

4. Perform all jumps with control.

Duration: Jump the series of boxes with 15 to 20 seconds rest between sets. Repeat 3 to 4 sets.

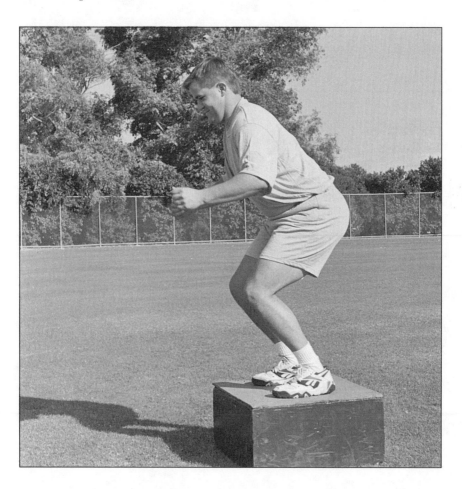

DEPTH JUMP AND SPRINT

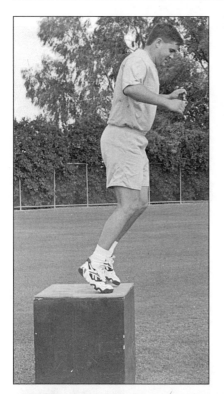

Focus: Teaching muscles to react forcefully from a negative contraction to a forceful positive contraction; quadriceps, gluteals, hamstrings, calf muscles

Procedure:

1. Drop off a box, landing with your knees slightly bent and feet about shoulder-width apart.

2. Immediately explode into a 10-yard sprint.

3. Jog back and repeat.

Repetitions: 5 to 8

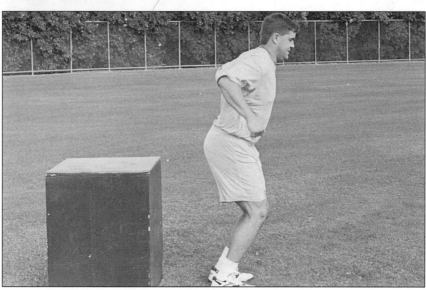

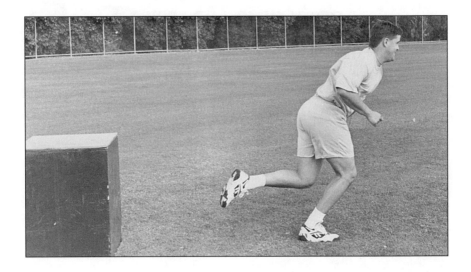

DEPTH JUMP WITH BASE STEAL

Focus: Teaching muscles to react forcefully from a negative contraction to a forceful positive contraction; quadriceps, gluteals, hamstrings, calf muscles

Procedure:

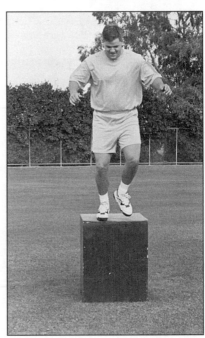

1.   Drop off a box landing with your knees slightly bent and feet about shoulder-width apart.

2.   Immediately cross over into a base-stealing position.

3.   Sprint for 10 yards.

4.   Jog back and repeat.

Repetitions: 5 to 8

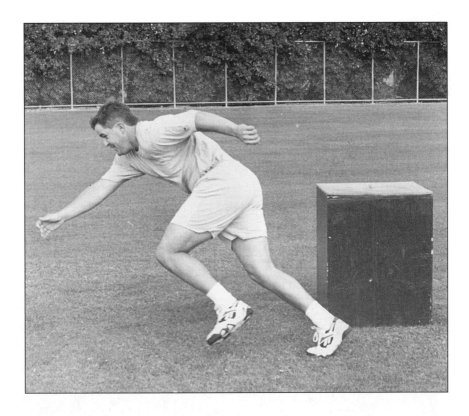

VELOCITY BELT BUILDER

One of the best training tools to improve and develop explosive balance, acceleration, vertical leap, and push-off power is the velocity belt builder. This apparatus consists of a platform with four latex tubes attached at the corners. The tubes attach to a belt and harness worn by the athlete, who stands in the center of the platform. A series of jumps and running drills can be performed using the velocity builder. The velocity builder is a great form of plyometrics and adds the convenience of supplying an excellent form of resistance while incorporating several different skill movements and jumps. You can find this piece of equipment through sports equipment dealers such as Triple Threat, Inc., in Tempe, Arizona (1-800-967-7011). Always follow velocity builder exercises with a series of drills of explosive jumps and running mechanics.

EXPLOSIVE VERTICAL JUMP

Focus:　Hamstrings, quadriceps, gluteals

Procedure:

1. In a squat position with your thighs parallel to the ground and your back upright, forcefully explode up, reaching high for the sky with your arms.

2. Land with your knees bent, back upright, and thighs parallel to the ground.

3. Gather and repeat immediately.

Repetitions:　Five to eight jumps immediately followed by the same number without the resistance bands. (Use same mechanics during contrast jumps.)

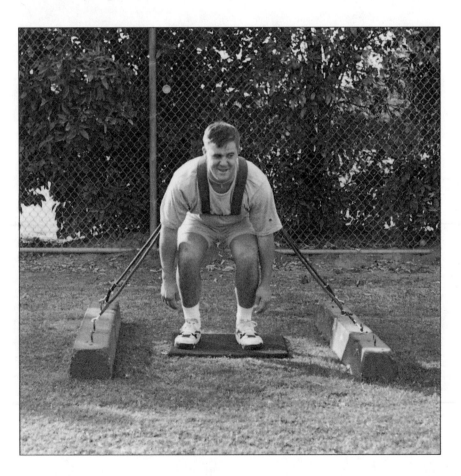

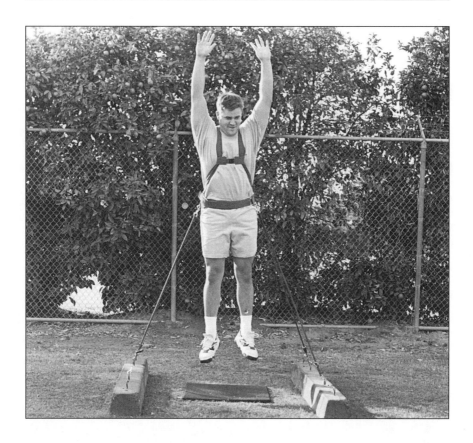

SIDE-TO-SIDE JUMPS

Focus: Building lateral explosion; quadriceps, hamstrings, gluteals, calf muscles

Procedure:

1. Stand on either side of a 6- to 12-inch hurdle or cone with your knee slightly bent and your feet about shoulder-width apart.

2. Laterally and explosively jump over cone or hurdle.

3. Land with knee bent and feet not quite shoulder-width apart.

4. Immediately jump back over cone or hurdle in the opposite direction.

5. Spend minimal time on the ground and continue the jumps in a rhythmic and controlled fashion.

Repetitions: 6 to 10 on each side

CHAPTER 9

MEDICINE BALL TRAINING

Medicine ball training, a form of plyometric training, can give the upper body a great explosive workout. Its multijoint movements can imitate baseball movements in various plays, angles, and motions. Medicine ball training is safe, inexpensive, and can be easily incorporated into many strength and conditioning programs. It takes up little space and is highly efficient in both team training and individual training.

Medicine balls usually range in weight from 2 pounds to 15 pounds. We recommend using 2- to 6-pound balls for beginners and drills requiring high repetitions, and 9- to 15-pound balls for more experienced players and lower body work. You can find medicine balls through sports equipment suppliers. You should incorporate a medicine ball training program into both your in-season and off-season training regimens. In season, work the program into your overall training schedule one to two times a week. In the off-season, increase the medicine ball routine to three to four times a week.

ADVANTAGES OF MEDICINE BALL TRAINING

Medicine ball training can improve your baseball game in five ways:

1. *By strengthening the core area.* Medicine ball training targets the core or center part of the body, which is the center of power and balance. The muscles making up the core consist primarily of the abdominals, the back muscles, the hip and gluteal muscles, and, to a lesser degree, the shoulders and upper legs. As we've mentioned, baseball is a rotational sport, and a strong core is essential for baseball players. It's involved in all facets of the game.

2. *By offering sport-specific training.* With the medicine ball you can closely imitate baseball movements with added resistance. Lunges and twists closely resemble routine movements in baseball, and throwing drills duplicate the throwing action as well.

3. *By developing explosiveness.* The medicine ball produces muscular contractions through the full range of the exercise. This develops the explosive ballistic firing patterns needed in your sport skill. To better understand explosiveness, think in terms of general, special, and specific strength. General strength requires the least amount of speed to perform specific sport skills and usually consists of weight-training exercises. These then would be the least explosive movements. Special strength more closely resembles actual performance, and specific strength is basically the actual performance coupled with resistance. Specific strength requires the greatest amount of speed. Since a medicine ball is a specific strength-training tool, training with a medicine ball helps develop explosive baseball movements.

4. *By building strength and power.* Training with the same movement patterns of your skill with the resistance of a medicine ball will help build the extra muscle mass and strength you need in baseball. Resistance with speed as you move the medicine ball through various angles and planes helps to enhance your athletic ability.

5. *By providing variability of resistance.* Medicine balls come in various weights and sizes, so you can choose the best weight and size for the skill movement you're working on. You can use heavier medicine balls for

the legs and more explosive movements and lighter balls for upper body exercises or those requiring higher repetitions. Remember that the heavier the ball, the greater the intensity.

TRAINING PROGRAM TIPS

1. Start slow—use general workouts that work the whole body.
2. Progress as you learn and master the movements.
3. Increase weight, intensity, and speed of movement after initial training base has been established.
4. Allow proper rest between sets. Start with 30 to 45 seconds and decrease the seconds as your cardiovascular and muscular endurance increases.
5. Start with five to eight exercises at about two sets of 8 to 20 repetitions. Eventually progress to five sets of 12 to 20 repetitions.
6. Variation helps to maintain interest and keep the body from adapting to the same workout.
7. Always have a good base and good balance when performing an exercise.
8. Consider the age and skill level of the athlete.
9. Have fun.

Use proper guidelines and some creativity to adapt programs to meet your needs. Always use a proper warm-up for the entire body to prepare for the workout.

SIDE LUNGES WITH MEDICINE BALL

Focus: Quadriceps, inner thigh, hamstrings, gluteals

Procedure:

1. Hold the medicine ball out in front of your chest and stand on the box.
2. Step off the box with your right leg and firmly plant your foot on the ground.

3. Lower your butt into a squat position until your thigh is parallel to the ground.

4. Drive back up forcefully using your right leg and return to the center of the box.

5. Repeat with the opposite leg.

Repetitions: 6 to 10 per leg

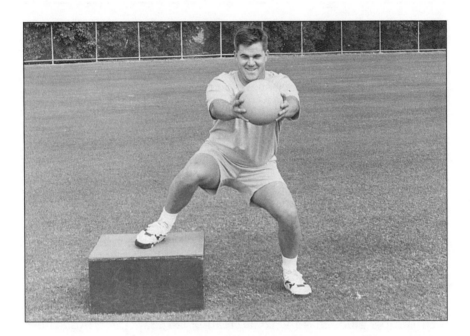

WOOD CHOP JUMPS

Focus: Hip flexors, gluteals, quadriceps, hamstrings

Procedure:

1. Start in a squat position holding the medicine ball extended out in front at knee level.

2. Simultaneously swing the medicine ball above your head and explode upward with a jump.

3. Land with your knees bent and return to the starting position.

4. Repeat.

Repetitions: 8 to 12, 2 to 3 sets

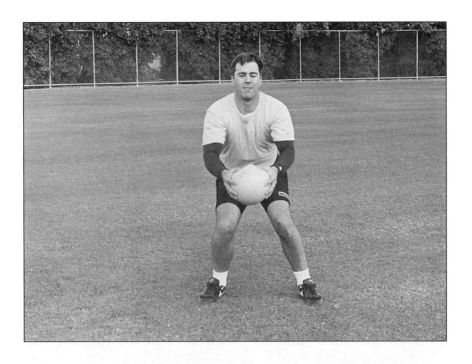

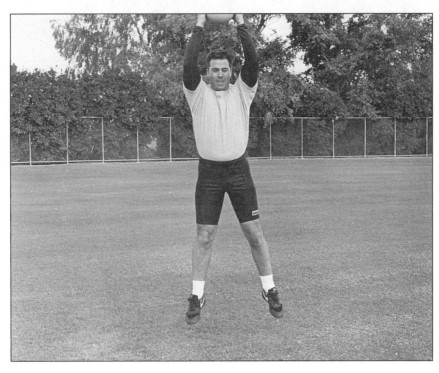

LUNGE WITH A TWIST

Focus: Quadriceps, gluteals, hamstrings, oblique and lower back muscles

Procedure:

1. Step forward with your leg in a lunge position, keeping your knee behind your toe and your chest behind your knee.

2. With the medicine ball, extend out in front of chest area with your lower right leg down and bent 90 degrees.

3. Twist the medicine ball to the side of your forward leg.

4. Return to the starting position and repeat the movement with your other leg.

Repetitions: 8 to 12 on each leg, 2 to 3 sets

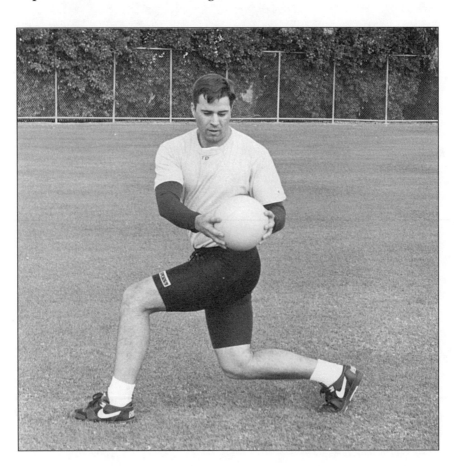

LEG SEPARATIONS WITH A LUNGE

Focus: Overall leg area and lower back

Procedure:

1.   Stand with your feet about shoulder-width apart and the medicine ball extended above your head.

2.   Step forward with your left leg into a lunge position, keeping your toe behind your ankle and your chest behind your knee.

3.   Simultaneously lower the medicine ball forward over your left toe. Perform this movement under control.

4.   Return to the starting position and repeat with your other leg.

Repetitions: 8 to 12, 2 to 3 sets

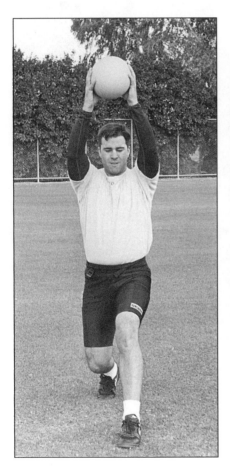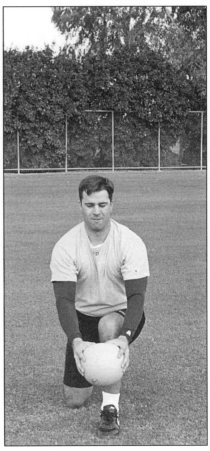

SCISSOR JUMPS

Focus: Speed power movement away from the center of your body; overall leg and hip region, gluteals

Procedure:

1. Start in standing position holding the medicine ball out in front of your chest.

2. Keeping your torso upright, cycle your leg forward in a lunge or straddle position.

3. Perform these movements in a continuous motion.

4. Stick in each landing for 1 second to ensure maximum intensity, proper mechanics, and balance.

Repetitions: 10 on each leg or timed intervals of 12 to 15 seconds, 2 to 3 sets

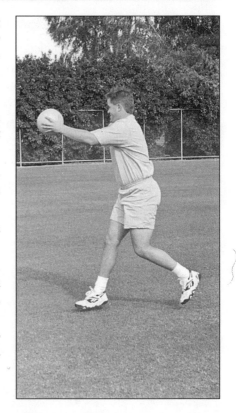

HIP TOSS

Focus: Obliques, abdominal wall, lower back, hip

Procedure:

1. Start laterally to your partner or target.

2. With the medicine ball at about hip level, twist the hip back along with the medicine ball.

3. Explode through with your hips and swing the ball through as you would with your swing or your hip rotation as you throw.

4. Reload and repeat movement on opposite side.

Repetitions: 10 to 12 on each side

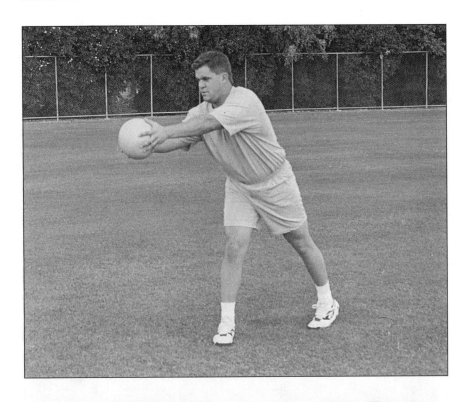

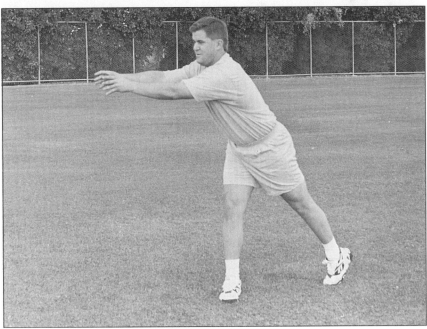

CHEST PASS

Focus: Chest and shoulder area

Procedure:

1. Standing, hold the medicine ball about chest level and step forward with either leg.

2. Forcefully push the ball away in a chest pass to a partner or up against a wall.

Repetitions: 8 to 12 or timed intervals of 10 to 15 seconds, 2 to 3 sets

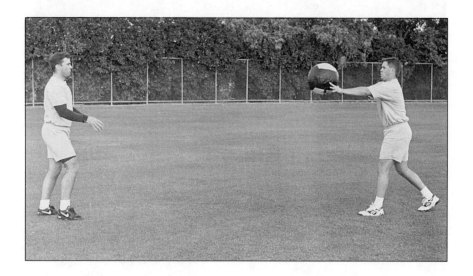

ONE-ARM PUTS

Focus: Shoulder, latissimus dorsi, lower back, hips

Procedure:

1. Standing laterally or in a throwing position, make sure your elbow is at shoulder level, the same as in throwing.
2. Load the medicine ball even with your ear.
3. Push the ball through in shot-put fashion, using your legs and back to reach out and get full extension.

Repetitions: 5 to 8, 2 to 3 sets

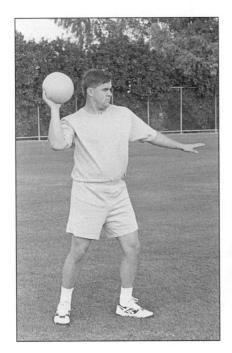

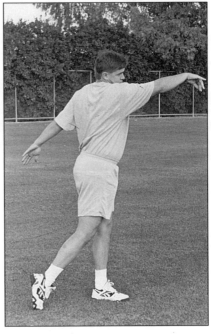

CHAPTER 10

COMBINATION TRAINING DRILLS

Adding variety to your workouts

will keep training challenging and keep your athletes' interest high over long training periods. These training drills blend strength, speed, agility, and plyometric components for highly explosive exercise that makes complete ballplayers. These drills also relate to skill-specific movements used on the baseball field. Complexity and intensity can be increased by adding resistance cords, reaction commands, and baseballs or tennis balls for hand-eye coordination.

Review each drill closely for a proper understanding of the patterns and mechanics and to ensure proper baseball movements are being used. These high-energy, explosive drills can be great additions to your training program. Be creative—make the drills fun, and consider making them competitive for team workouts. When first starting out, perform the drills for 10 to 15 seconds and gradually progress to 20 to 30 seconds as skill level increases. Add these drills into your regular conditioning program once or twice a week. In season, they are good time-savers because they cover speed, overspeed, and explosive training techniques. During team practices, you can include the drills as stations in a circuit type setting; individually, they can be performed as sets and repetitions.

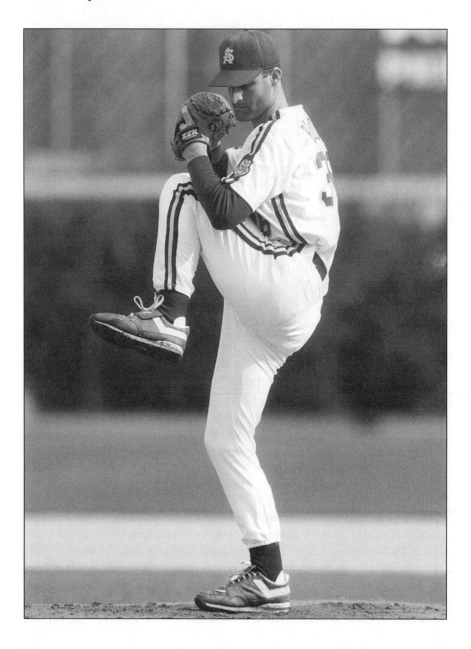

LINE DRILL

This particular drill involves only the use of a line, either on grass or a court. There are four different activities within the drill. Go through each drill one at a time, then repeat.

Focus: Quick feet, change of direction

Procedure:

1. Back and forth: Start with your toes perpendicular to the line so you can jump forward and backward over the line as fast as you can for 10 seconds.

2. Side to side: Stand parallel to the line so you can jump from side to side as fast as you can for 10 seconds.

3. Ali shuffle: Start with your feet apart and toes perpendicular to the line, then shuffle back and forth over the line as fast as you can for 10 seconds.

4. Criss-cross. Straddle the line. Once you start you'll go from feet apart to crossed over (with the right foot in front over the left), then immediately switch feet (left over right). Each time the feet will be on each side of the line, not on it, similar to the two-scissor movement.

Duration: 20 to 30 seconds, 2 to 3 times

FOUR-CORNER BASE STEAL

The four-corner base steal requires four cones placed in a square about 10 yards apart.

Focus: To work on the kind of explosive jump you need when stealing a base. Agility is also emphasized with the quick stops required and the sudden change of direction.

Procedure:

1. Moving counterclockwise to simulate the direction you travel when stealing a base, start on the outside of one of the cones and sprint to just past the next cone, being careful not to knock the cone down.

2. Stop and plant both feet in a "ready" position with your knees bent and torso up.

3. Cross over explosively, as you would to steal a base, and sprint just past the next cone. Plant your feet again and repeat this procedure all the way around the cones.

Duration: 20 to 30 seconds, 2 to 3 times. Up to four players can perform this drill at once.

COACHING TIPS

1. Look for good foot plant and body control.

2. Zone in on explosive crossover steps and maximum acceleration in the take-off.

3. Make sure all movements are positive. No popping up with your upper body or dropping your butt. Everything is directed toward the next cone.

FOUR-CORNER BASE STEAL

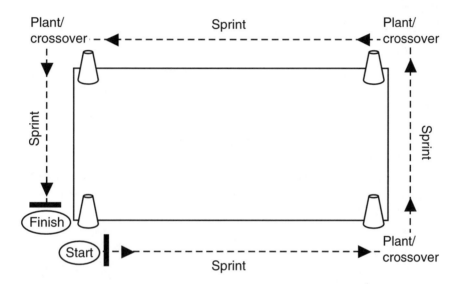

FOUR-CORNER BOX JUMPS

The four-corner box jump drill requires four plyometric boxes of three different heights—24, 18, 12, and 12 inches (you can double up on any of the heights). Place the boxes in a square about 15 yards apart (see the diagram).

Focus: To build explosive power while incorporating a skill movement

Procedure:

1. Start in front of one of the boxes. On command, jump onto the top of the box using mechanics the same as those you use in plyometric exercises. Knees should be slightly bent with your back straight and your butt tucked under your hips with good arm swing. Upon landing on top of the box, jump down using the same good mechanics.

2. Immediately break into a side-shuffle, maintaining a knees-bent, eyes-up position—as in a secondary lead during base stealing—to the next box.

3. As you approach each box, gather your momentum, plant both feet, and jump onto the box.

Duration: 20 to 30 seconds, 2 to 3 times. Up to four people can perform drill at once.

Variation: Box jump with base steal. Same format using break into a crossover step as you would stealing a base.

COACHING TIPS

1. Look for good mechanics on the jumps.

2. Make sure athletes are planting and jumping with two feet, with control.

3. When jumping down off of boxes, look for good athletic landing position. Knees should be slightly bent with back straight and butt tucked under hips.

FOUR-CORNER BOX JUMPS

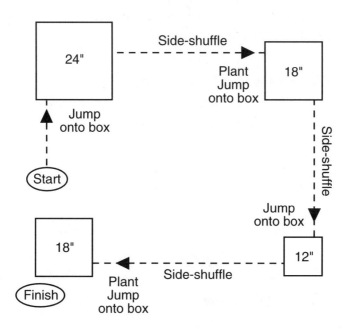

SPRINT SHUFFLE WITH CONE DRILL

This drill requires five cones set up in an inverted W shape (see diagram) with cones aligned 6 yards apart and 10 yards from cone to cone.

Focus: Change of direction, start and stop acceleration

Procedure:

1. Start at cone #1 and sprint to cone #2.
2. Plant your feet and then explosively shuffle to next cone.
3. Plant your feet and sprint to the next cone.
4. Shuffle through last cone.

Variations: Sprint-carioca-sprint or backpedal

Duration: 20 to 30 seconds, 2 to 3 times

COACHING TIPS

1. Look for good body control.
2. Stress explosive change of direction.
3. Time athletes and use their times for competition, fun, and improvement.

SPRINT SHUFFLE WITH CONE DRILL

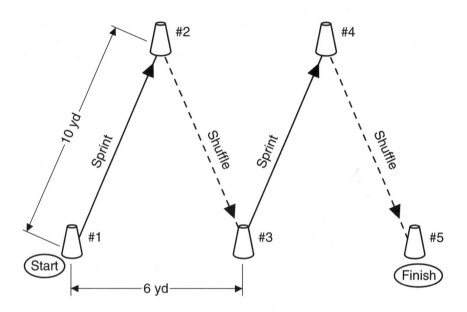

FIVE-POINT CONE DRILL

The five-point cone drill requires five cones set up as follows: place four cones in a square 10 yards apart. Place the fifth cone in the center of the square (see diagram). Using resistance belts and cords, make this drill an excellent combination of resistance, overspeed, agility, and acceleration.

Focus: Good change of direction and start and stop acceleration

Procedure:

1. Start at back left cone; if using a resistance belt and cord, make sure it's secure.
2. Sprint to the cone directly in front; with the cord, you have overspeed.
3. Plant and backpedal to the middle cone; with the cord you now have resistance.
4. Plant and sprint to the cone in front to your left.
5. Plant and backpedal to the cone behind you.
6. Plant and sprint forward through the last cone.

Duration: 20 to 30 seconds, 2 to 3 times

COACHING TIPS

1. Look for good acceleration and stops.
2. Stress good body control.
3. Look for controlled change of directions.

FIVE-POINT CONE DRILL

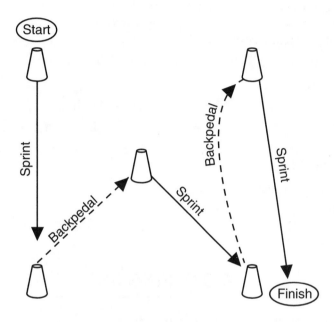

BALL PICKUPS CONE DRILL

Cone drill pickups are variations to work on quick change of direction and good body control. Follow the diagrams for placement of cones. Roll baseballs or tennis balls at designated targets.

Focus: To practice body control while performing your baseball skill

Procedure:

1. Shuffle laterally while fielding a ground ball.
2. Break and angle run to next cone while fielding a ground ball.
3. Plant your feet and shuffle back to the next cone while fielding a ground ball.
4. Change direction and repeat.

Duration: 20 to 30 seconds, 2 to 3 times

COACHING TIPS

1. Look for good acceleration and stops.
2. Stress good body control.
3. Look for controlled change of directions.

BALL PICKUPS CONE DRILL

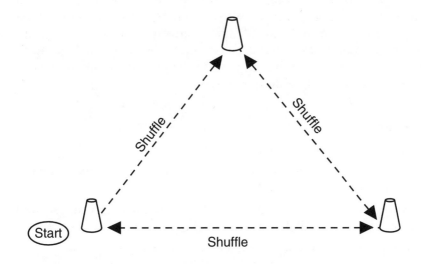

Field a ground ball at each cone

COMBINATION FOUR-CORNER WORK DRILL

The setup for the four-corner work drill requires four cones placed in a square 10 yards apart. You may use a variety of modalities with a different exercise at each cone. Players perform exercises with equipment at that cone and when finished sprint to the next cone to perform the next exercise. An example is given in the procedure below, but you may want to substitute different exercises.

Focus: Total body movement with change of direction

Procedure:

1. One to four players start at one of the cones.

2. Perform the prescribed exercise for the amount of time or repetitions prescribed.

3. When finished, sprint to the next exercise cone and repeat until you've completed all four stations.

Duration: 10 to 15 seconds, 2 to 3 times each corner

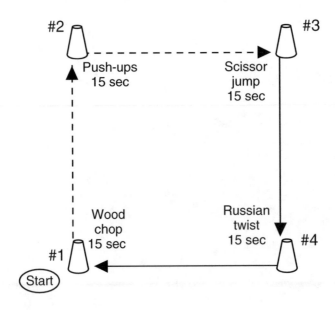

Move clockwise every 15 sec.

5-10-5 AGILITY DRILL

The 5-10-5 agility drill is designed to increase lateral speed and agility. Place two cones 10 yards apart. Place a third cone in the middle of the two cones at the 5-yard mark (see the diagram below).

Focus: To work on lateral explosive crossover steps and quick starts and stops in the opposite direction

Procedure:

1. Straddle the line with your body; clock starts upon forward movement.

2. Sprint to the right 5 yards and touch the line or cone with either hand.

3. Change direction and sprint 10 yards to your left and touch the line or cone.

4. Change direction and sprint past original starting place; clock stops.

Repetitions: Two times in each direction

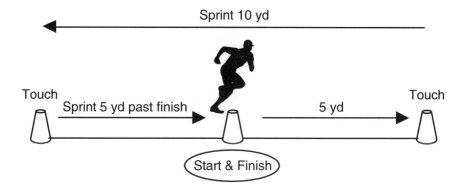

Sprint 10 yd

Touch

Touch

Sprint 5 yd past finish

5 yd

Start & Finish

CHAPTER 11

TRAINING PROGRAMS

Whether your conditioning

program succeeds will depend on the development of successive and consistent training sessions. When doing this, you need to address the needs of the specific individual or team. You can't generalize when assessing needs; the plan to "just get stronger" has been the downfall of many programs. Good intentions are usually not enough to build a successful program.

Rather, set specific goals and take a systematic approach to achieve them. Baseball players need to improve their strength, speed, agility, and endurance and reduce the risk of injury. Your program should be planned to achieve these goals. Weight training alone will not enhance all of these areas. Weight training combined with specific speed drills, agility and footwork drills, and explosive training exercises specific to baseball will increase the chances of obtaining your goal to be a better all-around baseball player.

Commit to improve your overall game. Your success starts in the weight room, gyms, basements, backyards, and playing fields. How good you want to be depends on how hard you're willing to work.

OFF-SEASON TRAINING

Tables 11.1 through 11.12 show a sample 12-week program for pitchers and position players during the off-season. As the principle of periodization suggests, the work levels are high, and the intensity increases each week. During this off-season phase, the players work on building overall strength, improving cardiovascular fitness, and sharpening their speed and ability for explosive action. Use this as a guideline to design a systematic conditioning program specific to your team's needs. The content of the actual practice sessions should be determined by the coach.

Table 11.1 Pitcher's Winter Training Schedule: Week 1

Tuesday		Thursday	
Flex/warm-up: 10 minutes		Flex/warm-up: 10 minutes	
Medicine ball:	Wood chops 2 × 10 Medicine ball toss 2 × 25 Scissor jumps 2 × 10	**Medicine ball:**	Wood chops 2 × 10 Medicine ball toss 2 × 25 Scissor jumps 2 × 10
Plyometrics:	Rapid box jumps 2 × 5 Side-to-side jumps 3 × 6	**Plyometrics:**	Rapid box jumps 2 × 5 Side-to-side jumps 3 × 6
Agility:	Side kick 2 × 15 sec Quick ladder 2 × 10 yd	**Agility:**	Side kick 2 × 15 sec Quick ladder 2 × 10 yd
Abdominals:	Russian twist 2 × 25 Crunch 2 × 25 Heel touches 2 × 25	**Abdominals:**	Russian twist 2 × 25 Crunch 2 × 25 Heel touches 2 × 25
Abdominals:	Crunches 2 × 25 Full crunch 2 × 25 Heel touches 2 × 25	**Abdominals:**	Crunches 2 × 25 Full crunch 2 × 25 Heel touches 2 × 25
Cardio work:	Sprints 2 × 220 yd 10-minute run	**Cardio work:**	Sprints 2 × 220 yd 10-minute run

Note: Mondays, Wednesdays, and Fridays are for weight training. See chapter 5.

Table 11.2   Pitcher's Winter Training Schedule: Week 2

Tuesday		Thursday	
Flex/warm-up: 10 minutes		**Flex/warm-up: 10 minutes**	
Medicine ball:	Hip toss 2 × 10 One-arm puts 2 × 10 Separation lunge 2 × 10 Lunge with twist 2 × 10	**Medicine ball:**	Hip toss 2 × 10 One-arm puts 2 × 10 Separation lunge 2 × 10 Lunge with twist 2 × 10
Plyometrics:	Rapid box jumps 2 × 5 Velocity builder 2 × 10	**Plyometrics:**	Rapid box jumps 2 × 5 Velocity builder 2 × 10
Agility:	Lateral box runs 2 × 12 sec Side kick 2 × 12 sec	**Agility:**	Lateral box runs 2 × 12 sec Side kick 2 × 12 sec
Abdominals:	Russian twists 2 × 25 Crunches 2 × 25 Heel touches 2 × 25	**Abdominals:**	Russian twists 2 × 25 Crunches 2 × 25 Heel touches 2 × 25
Cardio work:	Jump rope 12 minutes 10 × 60 yd sprints	**Cardio work:**	Jump rope 12 minutes 10 × 60 yd sprints

Note: Mondays, Wednesdays, and Fridays are for weight training. See chapter 5.

Table 11.3   Pitcher's Winter Training Schedule: Week 3

Tuesday		Thursday	
Flex/warm-up: 10 minutes		**Flex/warm-up: 10 minutes**	
Medicine ball:	Lunge with twist 3 × 10 Rapid chest pass 3 × 12 Wood chops 3 × 10 Hip toss 3 × 10	**Medicine ball:**	Lunge with twist 3 × 10 Rapid chest pass 3 × 12 Wood chops 3 × 10 Hip toss 3 × 10
Plyometrics:	Velocity build jumps 3 × 6 Sled pulls 3 × 20 yd Medicine ball toss/ sprint 3 × 50 yd	**Plyometrics:**	Velocity build jumps 3 × 6 Sled pulls 3 × 20 yd Medicine ball toss/ sprint 3 × 50 yd
Agility:	Side kick 3 × 15 sec Side tows 3 × 10 yd	**Agility:**	Side kick 3 × 15 sec Side tows 3 × 10 yd
Abdominals:	Jackknife sit-ups 3 × 25 Russian twists 3 × 25 Crunches 3 × 25	**Abdominals:**	Jackknife sit-ups 3 × 25 Russian twists 3 × 25 Crunches 3 × 25
Cardio work:	9-minute mile 5 × 60 yd sprints	**Cardio work:**	9-minute mile 5 × 60 yd sprints

Note: Mondays, Wednesdays, and Fridays are for weight training. See chapter 5.

Table 11.4   Pitcher's Winter Training Schedule: Week 4

Tuesday		Thursday	
Flex/warm-up: 10 minutes		**Flex/warm-up: 10 minutes**	
Medicine ball:	Separation lunges 3 × 10 Rapid chest pass 3 × 10 Seated twists 3 × 10 Scissor jumps 3 × 10	**Medicine ball:**	Separation lunges 3 × 10 Rapid chest pass 3 × 10 Seated twists 3 × 10 Scissor jumps 3 × 10
Plyometrics/ speed:	Weighted rope 3 × 15 sec Step-ups 3 × 15 sec Box jumps 3 × 15 sec	**Plyometrics/ speed:**	Weighted rope 3 × 15 sec Step-ups 3 × 15 sec Box jumps 3 × 15 sec
Agility:	Side kick 3 × 15 sec Side tows 3 × 10 yd	**Agility:**	Side kick 3 × 15 sec Side tows 3 × 10 yd
Abdominals:	Choose 3 exercises and do 3 sets of 25 each	**Abdominals:**	Choose 3 exercises and do 3 sets of 25 each
Cardio work:	Choose 2 cardio exercises	**Cardio work:**	Choose 2 cardio exercises

Note: Mondays, Wednesdays, and Fridays are for weight training. See chapter 5.

Table 11.5   Pitcher's Winter Training Schedule: Week 5

Tuesday		Thursday	
Flex/warm-up: 10 minutes		**Flex/warm-up: 10 minutes**	
Medicine ball:	Separation lunge 3 × 12 Side squats 3 × 12 Hip toss 3 × 12 One-arm puts 3 × 12	**Medicine ball:**	Separation lunge 3 × 12 Side squats 3 × 12 Hip toss 3 × 12 One-arm puts 3 × 12
Plyometrics/ speed:	Line touches (cord) 3 × 10 Resistance rows 3 × 4 Side-to-side jumps 3 × 10	**Plyometrics/ speed:**	Line touches (cord) 3 × 10 Resistance rows 3 × 4 Side-to-side jumps 3 × 10
Agility:	Side kick 3 × 15 Medicine ball shuffle 3 × 15	**Agility:**	Side kick 3 × 15 Medicine ball shuffle 3 × 15
Abdominals:	Choose 3 exercises and do 3 sets of 25 each	**Abdominals:**	Choose 3 exercises and do 3 sets of 25 each
Cardio work:	Choose 2 cardio exercises	**Cardio work:**	Choose 2 cardio exercises
Agility:	Side kick 3 × 15 Medicine ball shuffle 3 × 15	**Agility:**	Side kick 3 × 15 Medicine ball shuffle 3 × 15

Note: Mondays, Wednesdays, and Fridays are for weight training. See chapter 5.

Table 11.6   Pitcher's Winter Training Schedule: Weeks 6-12

Tuesday	Thursday
Flex/warm-up: 10 minutes	**Flex/warm-up: 10 minutes**
Medicine ball: Choose 4 exercises from medicine ball section and do 3 sets of 10 each	**Medicine ball:** Choose 4 exercises from medicine ball section and do 3 sets of 10 each
Plyometrics/ speed: Choose 3 plyometric/ speed exercises and do 3 sets of 10 each	**Plyometrics/ speed:** Choose 3 plyometric/ speed exercises and do 3 sets of 10 each
Agility: Choose 2 exercises from agility section and do 3 sets each of 15 seconds	**Agility:** Choose 3 plyometric/ speed exercises and do 3 sets of 10 each
Abdominals: Choose 3 exercises and do 3 sets of 25 each	**Abdominals:** Choose 3 exercises and do 3 sets of 25 each
Cardio work: Choose 2 cardio exercises adjusting duration up 5% each week	**Cardio work:** Choose 2 cardio exercises adjusting duration up 5% each week

Note: Mondays, Wednesdays, and Fridays are for weight training. See chapter 5.

Table 11.7   Position Player's Winter Training Schedule: Week 1

Tuesday	Thursday
Flex/warm-up: 10 minutes	**Flex/warm-up: 10 minutes**
Medicine ball: Hip toss 2 × 15 sec Wood chops 2 × 15 sec Scissor jumps 2 × 15 sec	**Medicine ball:** Hip toss 2 × 15 sec Wood chops 2 × 15 sec Scissor jumps 2 × 15 sec
Speed work: Arm swings 2 × 15 sec High knee runs 2 × 15 yd Resistance tows 2 × 3	**Speed work:** Arm swings 2 × 15 sec High knee runs 2 × 15 yd Resistance tows 2 × 3
Plyometrics: Choose 3 plyometric exercises from chapter	**Plyometrics:** Choose 3 plyometric exercises from chapter
Agility: Side kick 2 × 15 sec Quick foot ladder 2 × 15 yd Lateral box runs 2 × 15 sec	**Agility:** Side kick 2 × 15 sec Quick foot ladder 2 × 15 yd Lateral box runs 2 × 15 sec
Abdominals: Russian twists 2 × 25 Jackknife sit-up 2 × 25	**Abdominals:** Russian twist 2 × 25 Jackknife sit-up 2 × 25
Cardio work: Choose 1 exercise for 10 minutes (bike, run, stair climbing)	**Cardio work:** Choose 1 exercise for 10 minutes (bike, run, stair climbing)

Note: Mondays, Wednesdays, and Fridays are for weight training. See chapter 5.

Table 11.8   Position Player's Winter Training Schedule: Week 2

Tuesday		Thursday	
Flex/warm-up: 10 minutes		**Flex/warm-up: 10 minutes**	
Medicine ball:	Medicine ball toss 3 × 8 Hip toss 3 × 8 Rapid chest pass 3 × 8	**Medicine ball:**	Medicine ball toss 3 × 8 Hip toss 3 × 8 Rapid chest pass 3 × 8
Speed work:	Arm swings 3 × 15 sec Sled pulls 3 × 20 yd	**Speed work:**	Arm swings 3 × 15 sec Sled pulls 3 × 20 yd
Plyometrics:	Box jumps 3 × 5 Depth jumps with base steals 3 × 5	**Plyometrics:**	Box jumps 3 × 5 Depth jumps with base steals 3 × 5
Speed work:	Arm swings 3 × 15 sec Sled pulls 3 × 20 yd	**Speed work:**	Arm swings 3 × 15 sec Sled pulls 3 × 20 yd
Agility:	Side kick 2 × 12 sec Quick foot ladder 3 × 12 yd Lateral high knees 3 × 12 sec	**Agility:**	Side kick 2 × 12 sec Quick foot ladder 3 × 12 yd Lateral high knees 3 × 12 sec
Abdominals:	Choose 2 exercises and do 3 sets of 25 each	**Abdominals:**	Choose 2 exercises and do 3 sets of 25 each
Cardio work:	Choose 1 exercise for 15 minutes (bike, run, stair climbing)	**Cardio work:**	Choose 1 exercise for 15 minutes (bike, run, stair climbing)

Note: Mondays, Wednesdays, and Fridays are for weight training. See chapter 5.

Table 11.9   Position Player's Winter Training Schedule: Week 3

Tuesday		Thursday	
Flex/warm-up: 10 minutes		**Flex/warm-up: 10 minutes**	
Medicine ball:	Lunge and twist 3 × 10 One-arm puts 3 × 10	**Medicine ball:**	Lunge and twist 3 × 10 One-arm puts 3 × 10
Speed work:	Step-ups 3 × 8 Velocity builder arm kicks 3 × 10 Overspeed tows 5 × 20 yd	**Speed work:**	Step-ups 3 × 8 Velocity builder arm kicks 3 × 10 Overspeed tows 5 × 20 yd
Plyometrics:	Velocity builder jumps 3 × 6	**Plyometrics:**	Velocity builder jumps 3 × 6
Agility:	Slide board 3 × 15 sec Lateral box runs 3 × 15 sec	**Agility:**	Slide board 3 × 15 sec Lateral box runs 3 × 15 sec
Abdominals:	Choose 2 exercises and do 3 sets of 25 each	**Abdominals:**	Choose 2 exercises and do 3 sets of 25 each
Cardio work:	6 × 50-yd sprints	**Cardio work:**	6 × 50-yd sprints

Note: Mondays, Wednesdays, and Fridays are for weight training. See chapter 5.

Table 11.10   Position Player's Winter Training Schedule: Week 4

Tuesday		Thursday	
Flex/warm-up: 10 minutes		**Flex/warm-up: 10 minutes**	
Medicine ball:	Seated twists 3 × 10 Medicine ball toss 3 × 10 Separation lunges 3 × 10	**Medicine ball:**	Seated twists 3 × 10 Medicine ball toss 3 × 10 Separation lunges 3 × 10
Speed work:	Box runs 3 × 15 sec	**Speed work:**	Box runs 3 × 15 sec
Plyometrics:	Four-corner box jumps 2 × 20 sec Weighted rope 2 × 20 sec	**Plyometrics:**	Four-corner box jumps 2 × 20 sec Weighted rope 2 × 20 sec
Agility:	Side kick 3 × 15 sec Lateral shuffle w/ belt 3 × 15 sec Lateral high knees 3 × 15 sec	**Agility:**	Side kick 3 × 15 sec Lateral shuffle w/ belt 3 × 15 sec Lateral high knees 3 × 15 sec
Abdominals:	Choose 2 exercises and do 3 sets of 25 each	**Abdominals:**	Choose 2 exercises and do 3 sets of 25 each
Cardio work:	Sprints 2 × 220 yd 10-minute run	**Cardio work:**	Sprints 2 × 220 yd 10-minute run

Note: Mondays, Wednesdays, and Fridays are for weight training. See chapter 5.

Table 11.11   Position Player's Winter Training Schedule: Weeks 5-12

Tuesday		Thursday	
Flex/warm-up: 10 minutes		Flex/warm-up: 10 minutes	
Medicine ball:	Choose 3 exercises from medicine ball section and do 3 sets of 10 each	**Medicine ball:**	Choose 3 exercises from medicine ball section and do 3 sets of 10 each
Speed work:	Mechanics 3 × 10 Acceleration 3 × 8 Overspeed 3 × 5	**Speed work:**	Mechanics 3 × 10 Acceleration 3 × 8 Overspeed 3 × 5
Plyometrics:	Choose 3 exercises and do 3 sets of 8 each	**Plyometrics:**	Choose 3 exercises and do 3 sets of 8 each
Agility:	Choose 3 exercises and do 3 sets of 15 seconds each	**Agility:**	Choose 3 exercises and do 3 sets of 15 seconds each
Abdominals:	Choose 2 exercises and do 3 sets of 25 each	**Abdominals:**	Choose 2 exercises and do 3 sets of 25 each
Cardio work:	Choose 2 cardio exercises adjusting duration up 5% each week	**Cardio work:**	Choose 2 cardio exercises adjusting duration up 5% each week

Note: Mondays, Wednesdays, and Fridays are for weight training. See chapter 5.

IN-SEASON TRAINING

In-season training is a key component of overall body conditioning. This phase is designed to maintain the fitness, strength, and speed gains we achieved during the off-season. The combination of day-in, day-out playing takes its toll on the body. Maintaining a modified training program during the season helps your body stay strong for the duration of the season. At the same time, we should stress that in-season is not the time to try to gain strength but only to maintain the good body conditioning you need for day-to-day play.

During the in-season our primary emphasis is on our skill training, and other training is secondary. A two- to three-day strength maintenance program is more than adequate to minimize strength loss during the season (see tables 11.13 through 11.16). Any more than two to three days of excessive heavy lifting or overtraining promotes a loss of strength when coupled with day-in, day-out playing.

In-season training volume should be half of what you do during the off-season, and weight should be decreased by 30 to 40 percent. Keep intensity levels low. Following these guidelines will help to ensure that athletes are stronger over the course of the year and reduce their chances of injury. Following is an example of a six-week in-season/summer training program. Choose exercises that you feel are appropriate for you and/or your team and modify the routine accordingly. Keep routines short—about 20 to 40 minutes.

You can follow this type of training schedule week to week throughout the season. Choose different exercises to avoid monotony and adaptation of the body to the same routines. This is a great time of the year to incorporate the velocity builder, medicine balls, resistance cord, or speed runner routines. These tools provide good resistance and keep the body training with explosive movements. If you can't always get to the

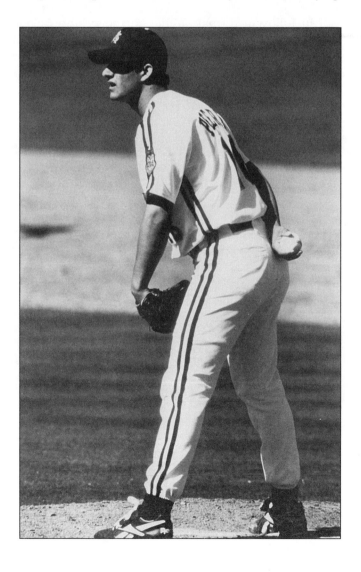

weight room during the season, the tools are doubly good. Note that your main work days are those opposite game days (Monday, Wednesday, and Friday in the examples below). Exercises listed on the other days can simply be incorporated into your stretching routine or light postgame work. Game day workouts should be done two to three hours before the game or, preferably, after the game.

The pitchers' running program should be monitored by the pitching coach. The running program should be scheduled with the previous week's work in mind, and if an off day has not been included during the week, Sunday should be considered an off day from running for the relievers.

Pitchers can follow a format similar to the position players. Base modifications on the pitching schedules of the starters. Emphasis for pitchers can be directed for more leg power and explosive work to help with endurance and leg strength over the season.

Table 11.12   Pitcher's In-Season Program: Week 1

Monday	Wednesday	Friday
Weights: Leg press 3 × 10 Dumbbell bench press 2 × 12 Biceps curls 2 × 12 Leg extensions/leg curls 2 × 12	**Combination:** Agility, plyometrics, medicine ball Velocity belt jumps 2 × 12 Lunge and twist 2 × 15 Rapid chest pass 2 × 10 Box lunges 2 × 15	**Weights:** Lat pulldown 2 × 15 Triceps extension 2 × 15 Lateral raise 2 × 12 Dumbell squats 3 × 10
Abdominal routine: 4 × 25	No abdominal routine	**Abdominal routine:** 4 × 25
Cardio work: Choice	**Cardio work:** Medicine ball throws Sprints 8 × 60 yd 15-minute run	**Cardio work:** Choice

Sunday	Tuesday	Thursday	Saturday
Off	Abdominals/cardio work	Abdominals/cardio work	Cardio work

Table 11.13 Pitcher's In-Season Program: Weeks 2-6

	Monday		Wednesday		Friday	
Weights:	Legs 3 × 10 Chest 2 × 12 Biceps 2 × 12 Leg extensions/leg curls 2 × 12		**Combination:**	Agility, plyometrics, medicine ball Plyometrics 2 × 12 Medicine ball 2 × 15 Agility 2 × 15 sec Combination drill 2 × 15	**Weights:**	Back 2 × 15 Triceps 2 × 15 Shoulders 2 × 12 Legs 3 × 10
Abdominal routine: 4 × 25			No abdominal routine		**Abdominal routine:** 4 × 25	
Cardio work:	Choice		**Cardio work:**	Choice	**Cardio work:**	Choice
Sunday		**Tuesday**		**Thursday**		**Saturday**
Off		Abdominals/cardio work		Abdominals/cardio work		Cardio work

Table 11.14   Position Player's In-Season Program: Week 1

	Monday	Wednesday	Thursday
Weights:	Leg press 2 × 12 Bench press 2 × 12 Biceps curl 2 × 12	Abdominals Forearms	Seated rows 2 × 15 Triceps pushdowns 2 × 12 Lateral raise 2 × 12 Leg curl/leg extension 2 × 12
Agility/speed:	Side kick 2 × 12 Box runs 2 × 12 sec Five-point cone drill 2 × 15 sec Mini-hurdle 4 × 12 yd		**Agility/speed:** Side kick 2 × 12 Box runs 2 × 12 sec Five-point cone drill 2 × 15 sec
Medicine ball:		Scissor jumps 2 × 15 sec Pullover throw/ medicine ball toss 2 × 10 Wood chop 2 × 10 Rapid chest pass 2 × 10	
Cardio work:	6 × 60-yd sprints	5 × 60-yd sprints	6 × 60-yd sprints

Sunday	Tuesday	Friday	Saturday
Off	Game	Game	Off

Table 11.15   Position Player's In-Season Program: Weeks 2-6

	Monday	Wednesday	Thursday
Weights:	Legs 2 × 12 Chest 2 × 12 Biceps 2 × 12	Abdominals Forearms	Back 2 × 12 Triceps 2 × 15 Shoulders 2 × 10 Legs 2 × 12
Agility/speed:	Lateral movement 2 × 12 Speed drill 2 × 12 sec Combination drill 2 × 15 sec Lateral/speed 4 × 12 yd		Lateral movement 2 × 12 Speed drill 2 × 12 sec Combination drill 2 × 15 sec Lateral/speed 4 × 12 yd
Medicine ball:		Scissor jumps 2 × 15 sec Medicine ball toss 2 × 10 Wood chop 2 × 10 Rapid chest pass 2 × 10	
Cardio work:	6 × 60-yd sprints	5 × 60-yd sprints	6 × 60-yd sprints

Sunday	Tuesday	Friday	Saturday
Off	Game	Game	Off

ABOUT THE AUTHORS

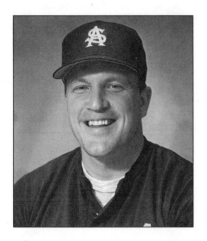

Patrick T. Murphy, who brought Notre Dame's baseball program from the bottom to the top during the seven seasons he served as head coach, is now piloting one of the country's premier college baseball programs at Arizona State. He is a member of the American Baseball Coaches Association and the NCAA Collegiate Baseball organization.

Jeff Forney is the strength and conditioning coach for the Arizona Diamondbacks. The author of several manuals, videos, and articles on strength and conditioning for baseball, he is a recognized leader in the study of explosive movements and their specific applications for baseball. He is a member of National Strength and Conditioning Association and American College of Sports Medicine.

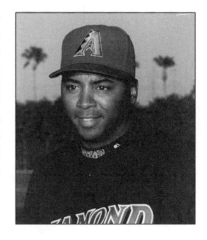